S0-BNH-758

An Atlas Of Dental Radiographic Anatomy

Myron J. Kasle, DDS, MSD

Howard R. Raper
Professor and Chairman of
Dental Radiology
Indiana University School of Dentistry
Indianapolis, Indiana

Third Edition

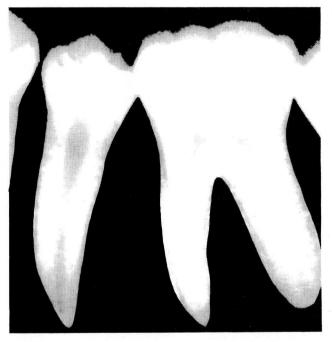

1989
W.B. SAUNDERS COMPANY
Harcourt Brace Jovanovich, Inc.
Philadelphia ▪ London ▪ Toronto ▪
Montreal ▪ Sydney ▪ Tokyo

W. B. SAUNDERS COMPANY
Harcourt Brace Jovanovich, Inc.

The Curtis Center
Independence Square West
Philadelphia, PA 19106-3399

Library of Congress Cataloging-in-Publication Data

Kasle, Myron J.

An atlas of dental radiographic anatomy.

Includes index.

1. Teeth—Radiography—Atlases.   2. Skull—Radiography—
Atlases.   I. Title.   [DNLM: 1. Radiography, Dental—
atlases.   WN 17 K19a]

RK309.K37 1990   617.6'07572   89–10186

ISBN 0–7216–5292–1

Editor: John Dyson
Designer: Paul Fry
Production Manager: Bill Preston
Manuscript Editor: Ruth Low
Illustration Coordinator: Lisa Lambert
Cover Designer: Michelle Maloney
Indexer: Diana Witt

An Atlas of Dental Radiographic Anatomy   ISBN 0–7216–5292–1

Copyright © 1990, 1983, 1977 by W. B. Saunders Company.

All rights reserved. No part of this publication may be reproduced or transmitted in any form or
by any means, electronic or mechanical, including photocopy, recording, or any information storage
and retrieval system, without permission in writing from the publisher. Library of Congress catalog
card number 89–10186.

Printed in United States of America.

Last digit is the print number: 9   8   7   6   5   4   3   2   1

TO MY WIFE, JUDY,
AND TO MY SONS, MICHAEL AND RICHARD

Preface

Time does fly when you're having fun. More than ten years ago, the first edition of the *Atlas* was published. It was intended then, as it is now, to help students of dentistry, dental hygiene, and dental assisting to understand the dental radiographic image.

It is not an easy task to interpret what is seen in a radiographic film. I hope the *Atlas* hits its intended mark of helping the reader to understand what is viewed.

The second edition of this book contained two new sections. Now, the third edition has been "beefed up" with the addition of some new materials in Film Artifacts and Technical Errors; Items Commonly Seen in Dental Radiographs; and the addition of a new section, Other Imaging Modalities.

A good book contains a fine index. It is the key to opening the door of knowledge. Use it well.

Personally, I think you'll refer to this *Atlas* for many years to come—many years beyond your formal schooling.

Good luck and good learning during those years of education, which if you think about it lasts your entire life.

MYRON J. KASLE

Acknowledgments

This third edition was developed with the assistance of some dedicated people.

Carol Ann Bauer typed the first two editions and was assisted with the third edition by Julie LeHunt. Gail F. Williamson, L.D.H., M.S., Assistant Professor of Dental Radiology at Indiana University School of Dentistry, helped with the collecting of many radiographs for all three editions. Dr. Angelo DelBalso, Dept. of Oral Radiology, Buffalo University School of Dentistry, Buffalo, New York; Dr. James G. Green, University of Nebraska School of Dentistry, Omaha, Nebraska; and Dr. Anoop Sondhi, private orthodontic practice, Indianapolis, Indiana, were all generous in sharing various radiographs.

Alana L. Barra and Mike Halloran of the Dental Art/Illustrations Department of Indiana University School of Dentistry provided the excellent photographs.

The W. B. Saunders Company is loaded with talented and highly dedicated people. I want to thank John Dyson, Senior Medical Editor, and Tom Stringer and Ruth Low, Copy Editors; Bill Preston, Production Manager; and their respective co-workers for their cooperation during the production of the Atlas.

MYRON J. KASLE

Contents

CONTENTS

SECTION ONE

INTRAORAL RADIOGRAPHS

Plate 1   MAXILLARY MOLAR REGION VIEW

A. Maxillary tuberosity
B. Floor of maxillary sinus
C. Zygomatic process
D. Maxillary sinus
E. Zygomatic arch
F. Shadow of soft tissue
G. Film identification dot
H. Coronoid process of mandible
I. Alveolar ridge
J. Retained roots
K. Pterygoid plate
L. Palatal root of permanent second molar
M. Mesiobuccal root of permanent first molar
N. Overlapping of tooth contacts
O. Floor of nasal fossa
P. Septum in maxillary sinus
Q. Hamulus or hamular process
R. Groove in maxillary sinus wall for superior alveolar nerve and vessels
S. Microdont
T. Distal surface of permanent second premolar
U. Artifact caused by fixer contamination

MAXILLARY MOLAR REGION VIEW   **Plate 1**

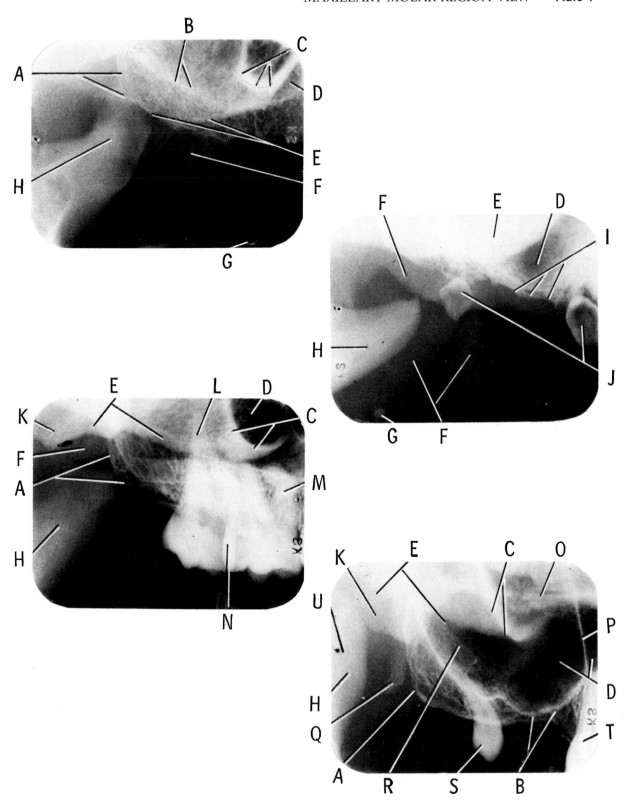

Plate 2   MAXILLARY MOLAR REGION VIEW

A.   Zygomatic process
B.   Maxillary sinus
C.   Posterior wall of maxillary sinus
D.   Hamular notch
E.   Maxillary tuberosity
F.   Coronoid process of mandible
G.   Lower border of zygomatic arch
H.   Palatal root of maxillary permanent first premolar
I.   Buccal root of maxillary permanent first premolar
J.   Distobuccal root of maxillary permanent first molar
K.   Mesiobuccal root of maxillary permanent first molar
L.   Dilacerated root of maxillary permanent second premolar
M.   Periapical radiolucency of maxillary permanent premolar
N.   Periapical radiolucency and buccal bone resorption of maxillary permanent first molar

MAXILLARY MOLAR REGION VIEW   **Plate 2**

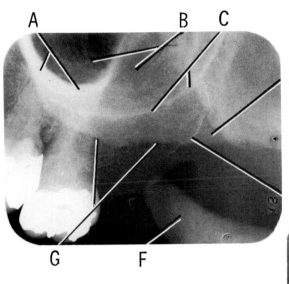

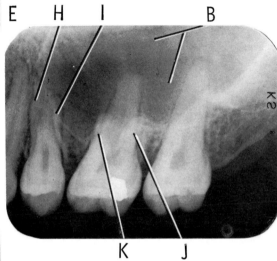

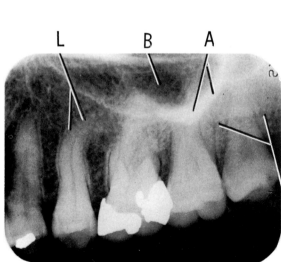

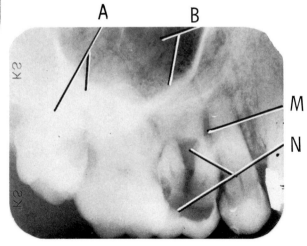

Plate 3   MAXILLARY MOLAR REGION VIEW

A.   Coronoid process of mandible
B.   Microdont
C.   Healed extraction site
D.   Maxillary sinus
E.   Unerupted maxillary permanent third molar
F.   Follicle of maxillary permanent third molar
G.   Hamulus—medial pterygoid plate
H.   Zygomatic process

MAXILLARY MOLAR REGION VIEW   **Plate 3**

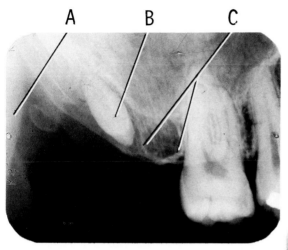

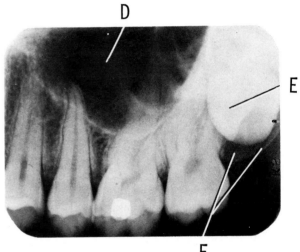

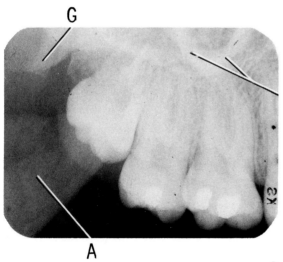

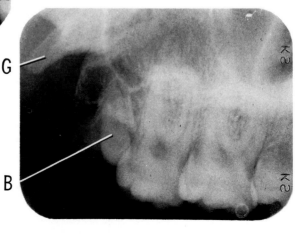

Plate 4   MAXILLARY MOLAR REGION VIEW

A.   Lower border of zygomatic arch
B.   Maxillary sinus
C.   Maxillary tuberosity
D.   Sclerotic bone
E.   Maxillary sinus depression
F.   Zygomatic process
G.   Lateral pterygoid plate
H.   Hamulus—medial pterygoid plate
I.   Coronoid process of mandible
J.   Film identification dot
K.   Floor of maxillary sinus
L.   Nutrient canal in maxillary sinus wall
M.   Soft tissue covering maxillary tuberosity
N.   Sequestrum from previous extraction

MAXILLARY MOLAR REGION VIEW   **Plate 4**

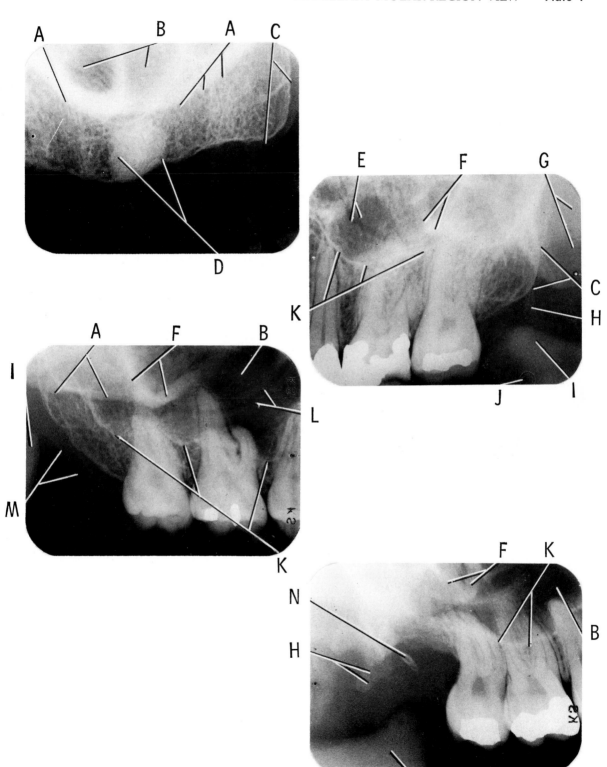

Plate 5   MAXILLARY MOLAR REGION VIEW

A.   Nasal fossa
B.   Floor of nasal fossa
C.   Maxillary sinus
D.   Floor of maxillary sinus
E.   Mesiobuccal root of maxillary permanent first molar
F.   Distobuccal root of maxillary permanent first molar
G.   Palatal root of maxillary permanent first molar
H.   Endodontic treatment in root of maxillary permanent second premolar
I.   Recurrent caries under gold crown of maxillary permanent first molar
J.   Coronoid process of mandible
K.   Film identification dot
L.   Zygomatic process
M.   Nutrient canal in maxillary sinus wall

MAXILLARY MOLAR REGION VIEW   **Plate 5**

Plate 6   MAXILLARY MOLAR REGION VIEW

A.   Lateral pterygoid plate
B.   Hamulus—medial pterygoid plate
C.   Film identification dot
D.   Coronoid process of mandible
E.   Maxillary sinus
F.   Zygomatic process
G.   Soft tissue shadow
H.   Thin plate of bone distal to maxillary third molar
I.   Impacted maxillary permanent third molar
J.   Soft tissue over maxillary third molar
K.   Impacted supernumerary molar
L.   Chrome steel orthodontic band

MAXILLARY MOLAR REGION VIEW   **Plate 6**

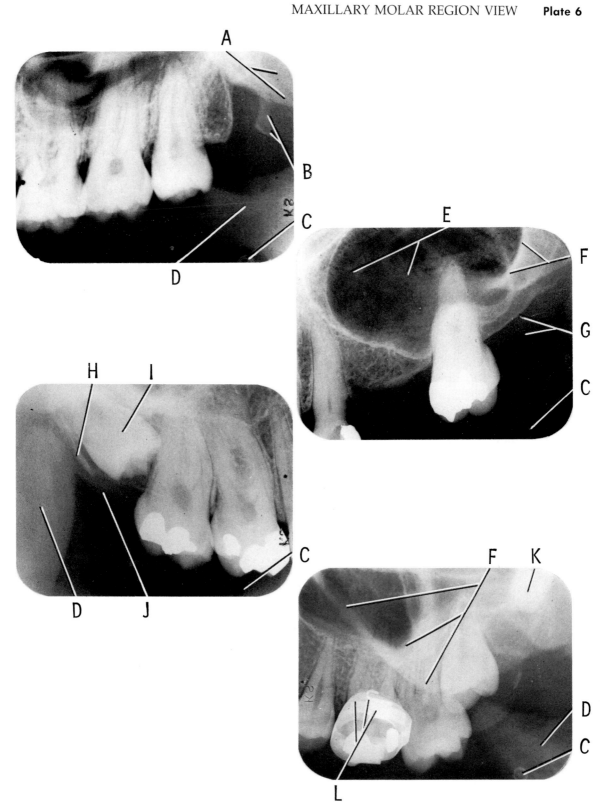

Plate 7   MAXILLARY PREMOLAR REGION VIEW

A.   Unerupted maxillary permanent first molar
B.   Unerupted maxillary permanent second premolar
C.   Unerupted maxillary permanent first premolar
D.   Unerupted maxillary permanent canine
E.   Partially resorbed root of maxillary primary canine
F.   Maxillary primary first molar
G.   Maxillary primary second molar
H.   Radiolucent resin restoration
I.   Radiopaque metallic lingual restoration
J.   Endodontically treated maxillary permanent first premolar with retrograde metal restoration
K.   Gold post and core restoration
L.   Floor of nasal fossa
M.   Buccal root of maxillary permanent first premolar
N.   Palatal root of maxillary permanent first premolar
O.   Nutrient canal in maxillary sinus wall

MAXILLARY PREMOLAR REGION VIEW   **Plate 7**

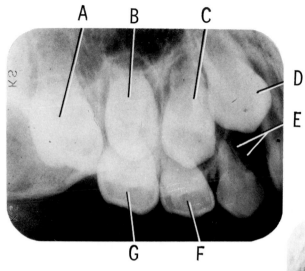

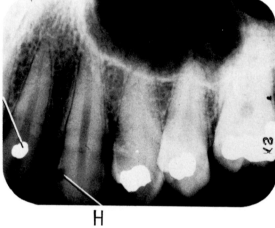

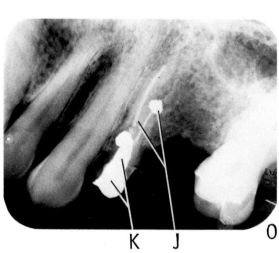

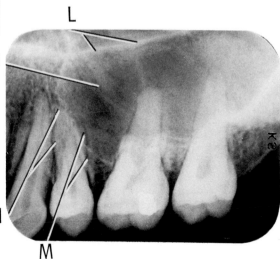

Plate 8   MAXILLARY PREMOLAR REGION VIEW

A. Zygomatic process
B. Maxillary sinus
C. Oroantral fistula
D. Supernumerary tooth
E. Film crease
F. Septum in maxillary sinus
G. Sclerosed pulp chambers
H. Resorbed bone of edentulous arch
I. Floor of nasal fossa
J. Cusp of mandibular permanent first molar
K. Maxillary primary second molar
L. Maxillary primary first molar
M. Maxillary primary canine

MAXILLARY PREMOLAR REGION VIEW   **Plate 8**

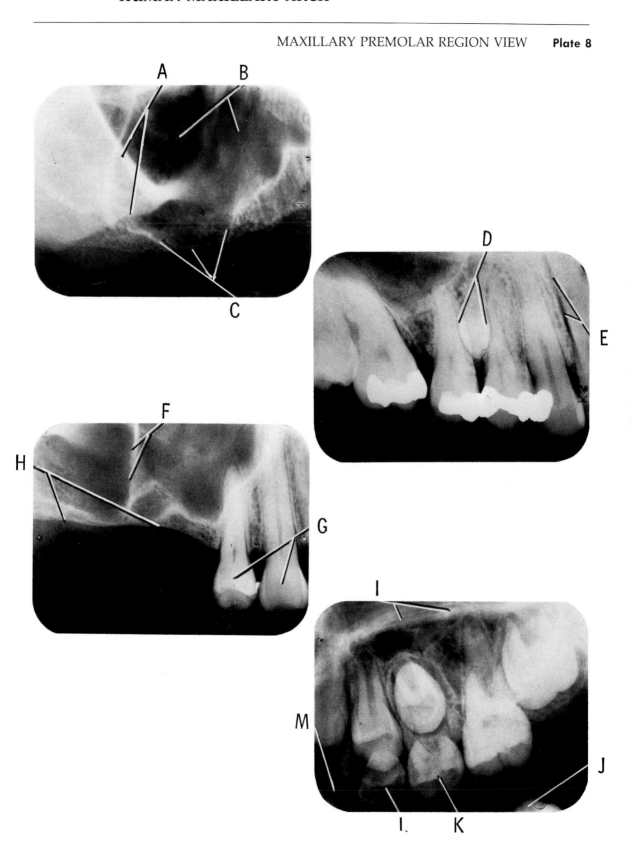

Plate 9   MAXILLARY PREMOLAR REGION VIEW

A.   Maxillary sinus
B.   Zygoma
C.   Groove of nutrient canal in maxillary sinus
D.   Remnant of retained root tip
E.   Cervical burnout (adumbration)
F.   Septum in maxillary sinus
G.   Nasolabial fold
H.   Microdont
I.   Gold pontics
J.   Gold crown abutments

MAXILLARY PREMOLAR REGION VIEW   **Plate 9**

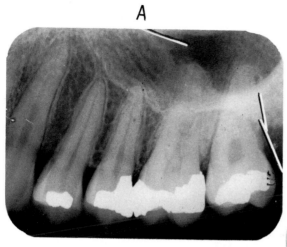

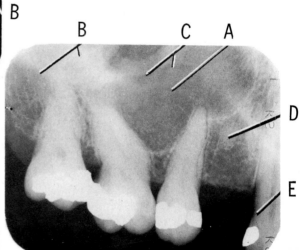

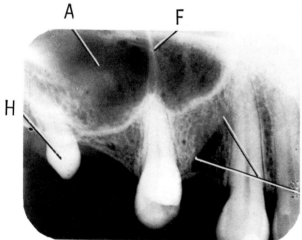

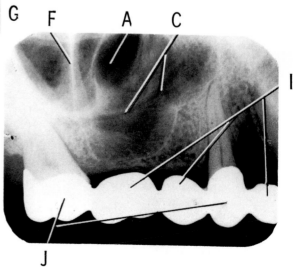

Plate 10   MAXILLARY PREMOLAR REGION VIEW

A.   Floor of maxillary sinus
B.   Maxillary sinus
C.   Zygomatic process
D.   Carious lesions
E.   Septa in maxillary sinus
F.   Palatal root of maxillary permanent first molar
G.   Lower border of zygomatic arch
H.   Periapical radiolucency of mesial root, maxillary permanent first molar
I.   Gold crown abutment of maxillary permanent canine
J.   Gold pontics for maxillary bridge
K.   Gold crown abutment of maxillary permanent first molar
L.   Floor of nasal fossa

MAXILLARY PREMOLAR REGION VIEW   **Plate 10**

Plate 11   MAXILLARY PREMOLAR-MOLAR REGION VIEW

    A.   Maxillary sinus septum
    B.   Palatal roots
    C.   Maxillary tuberosity
    D.   Area of bone resorption
    E.   Heavy calculus deposits
    F.   Compound odontoma
    G.   Palatal cusp of maxillary permanent first premolar

MAXILLARY PREMOLAR-MOLAR REGION VIEW   **Plate 11**

Plate 12   MAXILLARY CANINE REGION VIEW

A.   Maxillary sinus
B.   Bone septum separating nasal fossa and maxillary sinus
C.   Nasal fossa
D.   Nasolabial fold
E.   Shadow of nose
F.   Cement base
G.   Resin restoration
H.   Gold post and core in endodontically treated tooth
I.   Periapical radiolucency in infected tooth
J.   Pulpally exposed tooth

MAXILLARY CANINE REGION VIEW   **Plate 12**

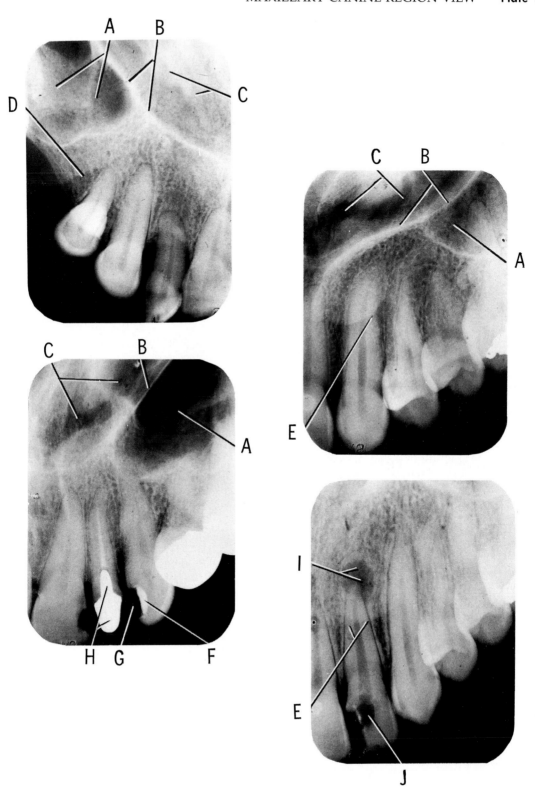

Plate 13   MAXILLARY CANINE REGION VIEW

A.   Maxillary sinus
B.   Bone septum between nasal fossa and maxillary sinus
C.   Nasal fossa
D.   Radiolucent resin restorations
E.   Maxillary primary canine
F.   Maxillary primary first molar
G.   Nasal septum
H.   Carious lesion in maxillary permanent first premolar
I.   Radiopaque cement
J.   Crown prepared for jacket crown restoration
K.   Metal tubing post placed in pulp canal
L.   Carious lesion in maxillary permanent central incisor
M.   Periapical lesion due to metal tubing in pulp canal

MAXILLARY CANINE REGION VIEW   **Plate 13**

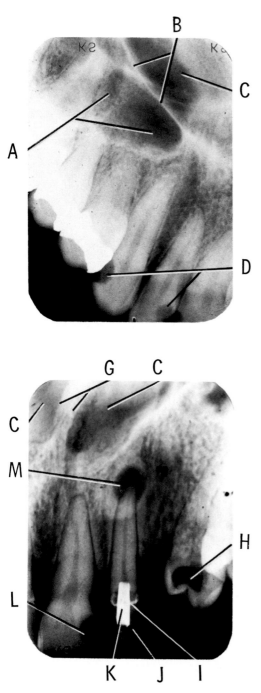

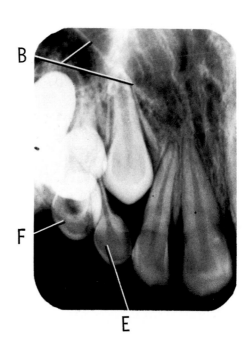

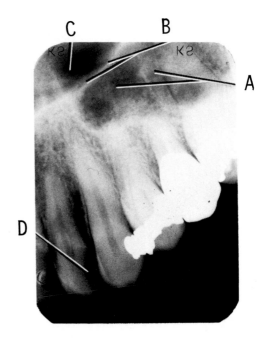

Plate 14   MAXILLARY CANINE REGION VIEW

A.   Bone separating nasal fossa and maxillary sinus
B.   Nasal fossa
C.   Alveolus of recently extracted maxillary permanent lateral incisor
D.   Alveolus of recently extracted maxillary permanent central incisor
E.   Maxillary permanent canine
F.   Buccal cusp of maxillary permanent first premolar
G.   Palatal cusp of maxillary permanent first premolar
H.   Maxillary permanent second premolar
I.   Shadow of soft tissue of nose
J.   Floor of maxillary sinus
K.   Maxillary sinus
L.   Maxillary permanent central incisors
M.   Transposed maxillary permanent first premolar
N.   Transposed maxillary permanent canine
O.   Metal restorations
P.   Follicle of maxillary permanent canine
Q.   Incisive foramen
R.   Unerupted maxillary permanent canine
S.   Maxillary permanent lateral incisor
T.   Palatal cusp of maxillary permanent second premolar
U.   Buccal cusp of maxillary permanent second premolar
V.   Shadow of maxillary permanent first molar
W.   Septum in maxillary sinus
X.   Resin restorations
Y.   Film identification dot

MAXILLARY CANINE REGION VIEW   **Plate 14**

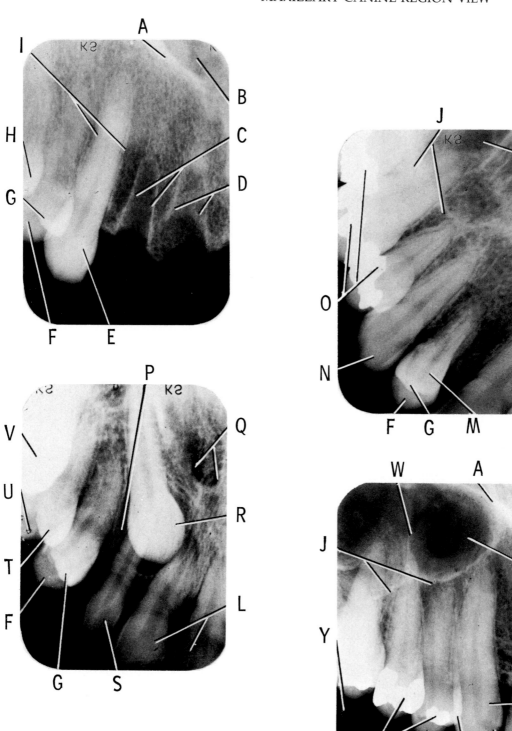

Plate 15   MAXILLARY CANINE REGION VIEW

A.	Nasal fossa
B.	Floor of nasal fossa
C.	Maxillary sinus
D.	Floor of maxillary sinus
E.	Buccal root of maxillary permanent first premolar
F.	Palatal root of maxillary permanent first premolar
G.	Buccal cusp of maxillary permanent first premolar
H.	Resin restoration
I.	Cement base
J.	Metallic lingual restoration
K.	Film identification dot
L.	Shadow of maxillary permanent first premolar
M.	Overlapping contacts
N.	Periapical radiolucency around maxillary permanent first premolar
O.	Carious lesion
P.	Periapical radiolucency around maxillary permanent lateral incisor
Q.	Palatal cusp of maxillary permanent second premolar
R.	Palatal cusp of maxillary permanent first premolar
S.	Resorbed root of maxillary permanent lateral incisor

MAXILLARY CANINE REGION VIEW   **Plate 15**

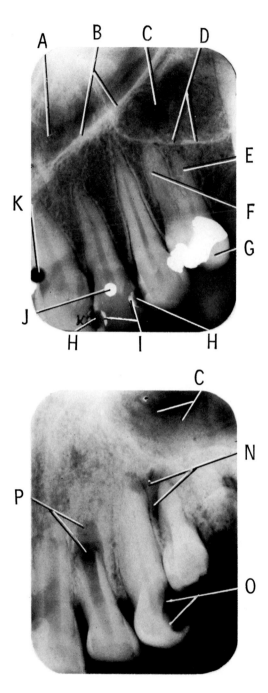

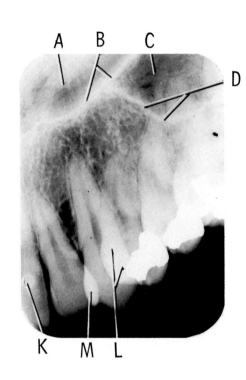

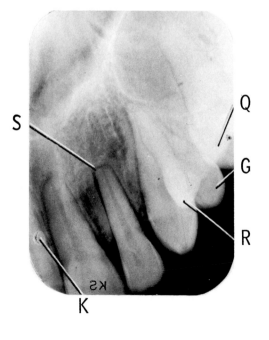

Plate 16   MAXILLARY INCISOR REGION VIEW

A.   Maxillary primary lateral incisor
B.   Unerupted maxillary permanent lateral incisor
C.   Developing root of erupting maxillary permanent central incisor
D.   Nasal fossa
E.   Nasal septum
F.   Median palatal suture
G.   Crowns of maxillary primary central incisors with resorbed roots
H.   Anterior nasal spine
I.   Mesiodens
J.   Opening made on lingual side of tooth for attempted endodontic treatment
K.   Erosion
L.   Endodontic filling material
M.   Silver alloy retrograde filling
N.   Resin restorations

MAXILLARY INCISOR REGION VIEW   **Plate 16**

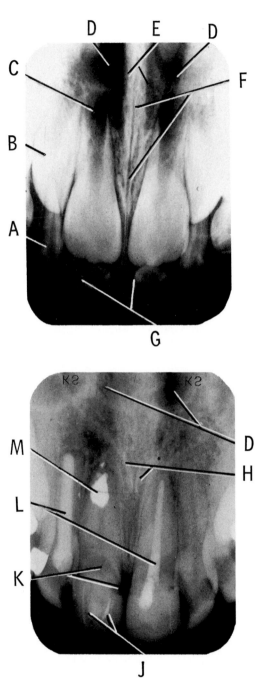

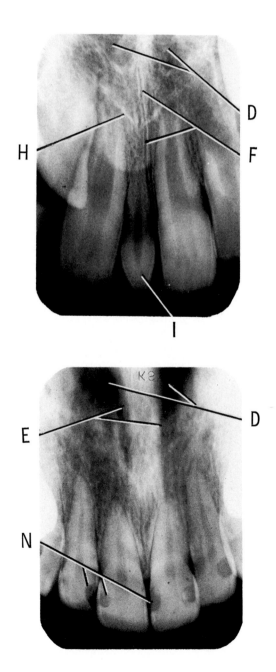

Plate 17   MAXILLARY INCISOR REGION VIEW

A.	Nasal fossa
B.	Nasal septum
C.	Anterior nasal spine
D.	Incisive foramen
E.	Lip line
F.	Lingual metal restoration
G.	Median palatal suture
H.	Film identification dot
I.	Anterior extent of maxillary sinus
J.	Carious lesion
K.	Gold pontic
L.	Gold crown restoration
M.	Surgical defect
N.	Soft tissue of nose

MAXILLARY INCISOR REGION VIEW   **Plate 17**

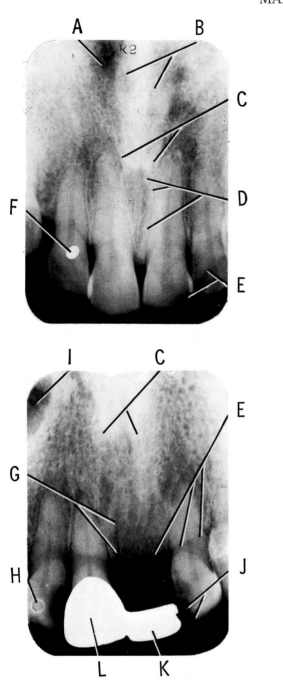

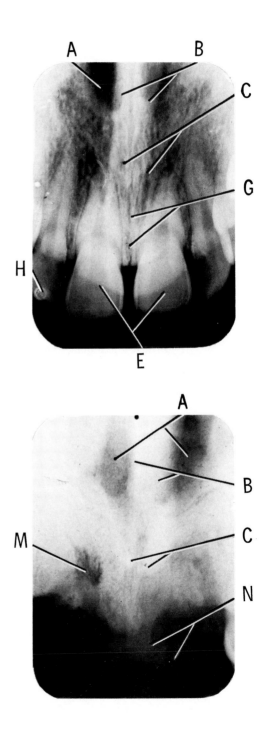

Plate 18   MAXILLARY INCISOR REGION VIEW

A.   Unerupted maxillary permanent canine
B.   Nasal septum
C.   Radiolucent line indicating cervical area and bone level
D.   Shadow of soft tissue of nose
E.   Gold pontics of anterior bridge
F.   Nasal fossa
G.   Supernumerary teeth
H.   Unerupted maxillary permanent lateral incisor
I.   Unerupted maxillary permanent central incisor
J.   Maxillary primary lateral incisor
K.   Maxillary primary central incisor

MAXILLARY INCISOR REGION VIEW   **Plate 18**

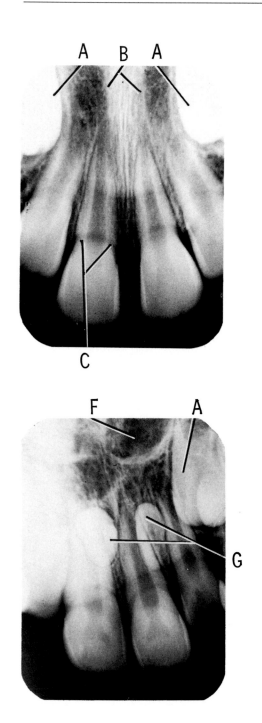

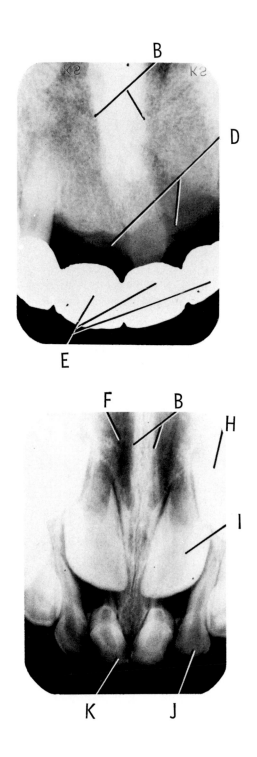

Plate 19   MAXILLARY INCISOR REGION VIEW

A.   Nasal fossa
B.   Anterior nasal spine
C.   Carious lesion
D.   Median palatal suture
E.   Incisive nerve foramen
F.   Periapical lesion
G.   Carious lesion involving pulp chamber
H.   Shadow of lip line
I.   Supernumerary tooth (mesiodens)
J.   Nasal septum
K.   Developing roots of maxillary permanent central incisors
L.   Crown remnants of maxillary primary lateral incisors

MAXILLARY INCISOR REGION VIEW   **Plate 19**

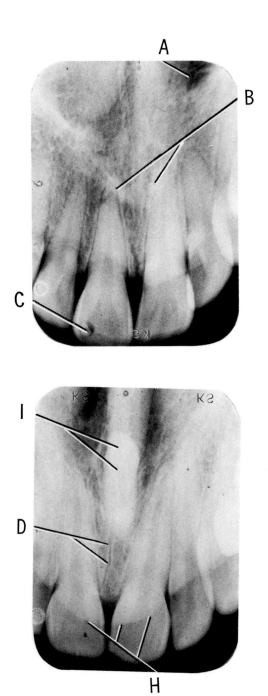

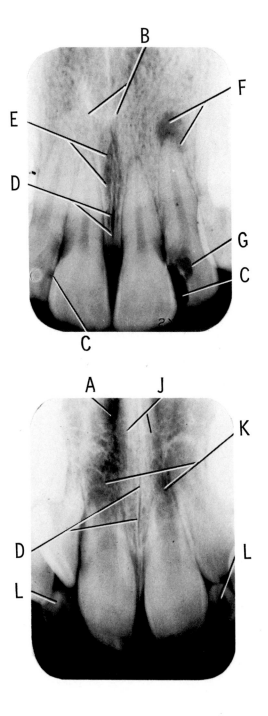

Plate 20   MAXILLARY INCISOR REGION VIEW

A.   Impacted maxillary permanent central incisor
B.   Nasal fossae
C.   Incisal attrition
D.   Resorbed root
E.   Gold post and core of endodontically treated maxillary permanent central incisors
F.   Reinforcing wire under resin restoration replacing fractured incisal edge
G.   Overlapping of maxillary permanent lateral and central incisors
H.   Crown fracture of maxillary permanent central incisor
I.   Shadow of lip line

MAXILLARY INCISOR REGION VIEW   **Plate 20**

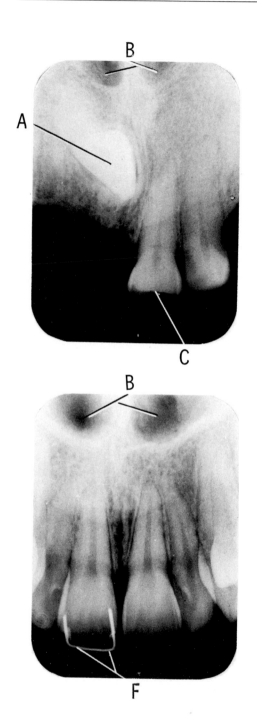

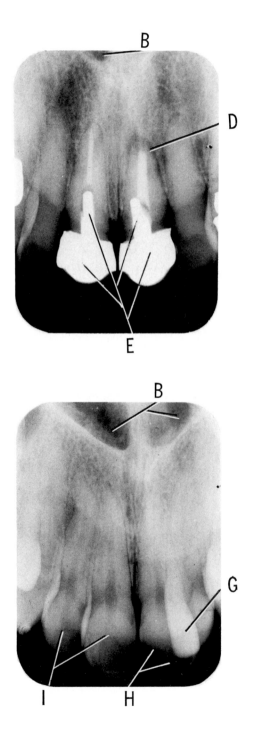

Plate 21   MAXILLARY INCISOR REGION VIEW

A.	Nasal conchae in nasal fossae
B.	Nasal fossae
C.	Anterior nasal spine
D.	Shadow of lip line
E.	Nasal septum
F.	Incisive nerve foramen
G.	Area of missing anterior restoration
H.	Carious lesion
I.	Median palatal suture
J.	Resorbed roots
K.	Resin restoration

MAXILLARY INCISOR REGION VIEW   **Plate 21**

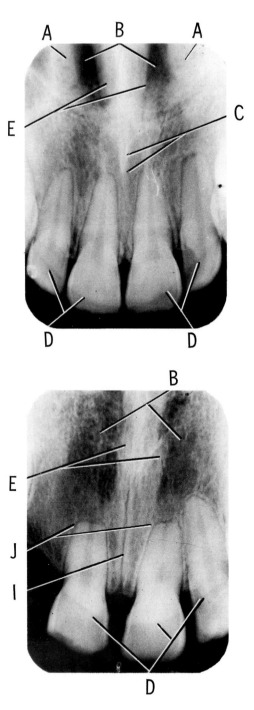

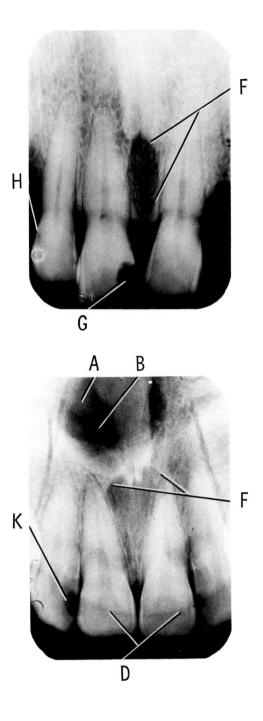

Plate 22   MAXILLARY INCISOR REGION VIEW

A.   Nasal fossa
B.   Nasal septum
C.   Film crease
D.   Impacted maxillary permanent canine
E.   Rubber material around metal film holder
F.   Metal film holder
G.   Soft tissue of nose
H.   Zinc oxide temporary restoration
I.   Anterior nasal spine
J.   Cement bases under resin restorations
K.   Carious lesion

MAXILLARY INCISOR REGION VIEW   **Plate 22**

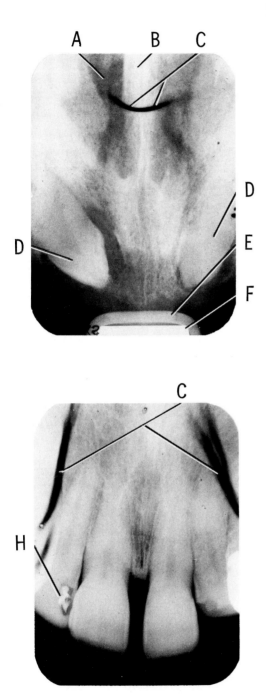

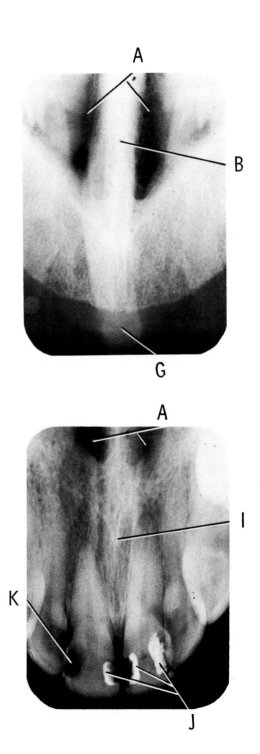

Plate 23   MANDIBULAR MOLAR REGION VIEW

A.   Mandibular canal
B.   Film identification dot
C.   External oblique ridge
D.   Cervical burnout (adumbration)
E.   Enamel pearl
F.   Internal oblique ridge
G.   Overhanging restoration
H.   Radiolucent normal bone area

MANDIBULAR MOLAR REGION VIEW   **Plate 23**

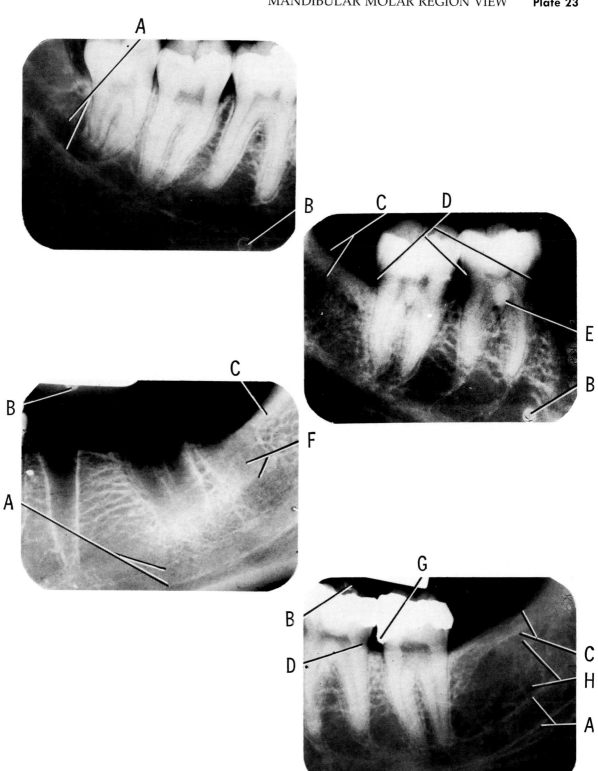

Plate 24   MANDIBULAR MOLAR REGION VIEW

A. Recurrent caries
B. Area of bone resorption
C. Fused roots
D. Dilacerated root
E. Mandibular canal
F. Healing extraction site

MANDIBULAR MOLAR REGION VIEW   **Plate 24**

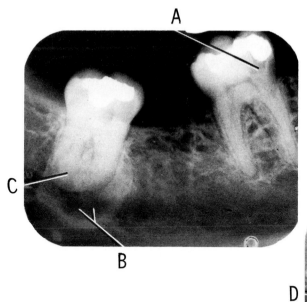

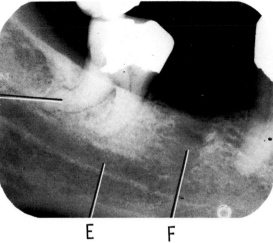

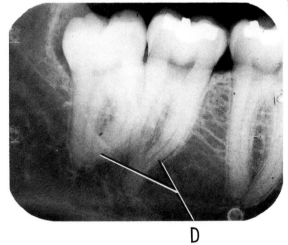

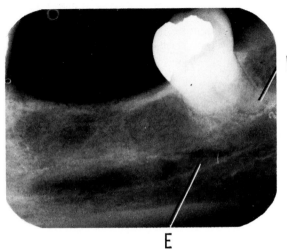

Plate 25   MANDIBULAR MOLAR REGION VIEW

A.   Pulp stone
B.   Retained root fragments
C.   Radiolucency indicating bone resorption
D.   Radiolucency indicating bone destruction due to periodontal disease
E.   Film identification dot
F.   Mandibular canal
G.   External oblique ridge
H.   Enamel pearl
I.   Cortical bone of inferior border of mandible
J.   Healing extraction site
K.   Tooth crown destruction due to caries
L.   Bone overlying developing permanent third molar
M.   Developing permanent third molar in follicle
N.   Early calcification of bifurcation of permanent third molar
O.   Periapical bone loss due to carious lesion
P.   Cervical burnout (adumbration)

MANDIBULAR MOLAR REGION VIEW   **Plate 25**

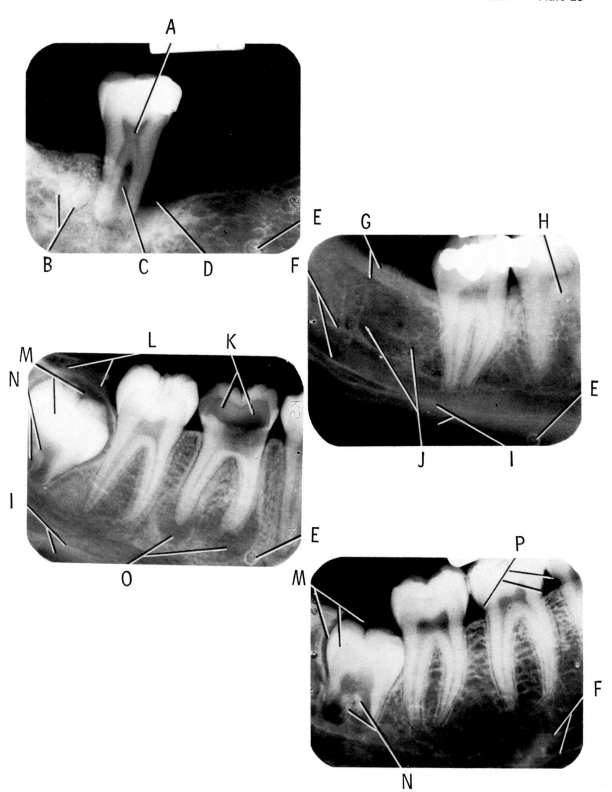

Plate 26   MANDIBULAR MOLAR REGION VIEW

A.   Lamina dura of tooth follicle
B.   Developing mandibular permanent third molar in follicle
C.   Alveolar bone level
D.   Developing roots of mandibular permanent second molar
E.   Horizontal developing mandibular permanent third molar
F.   Overhanging restoration
G.   Horizontally impacted mandibular permanent third molar

MANDIBULAR MOLAR REGION VIEW   **Plate 26**

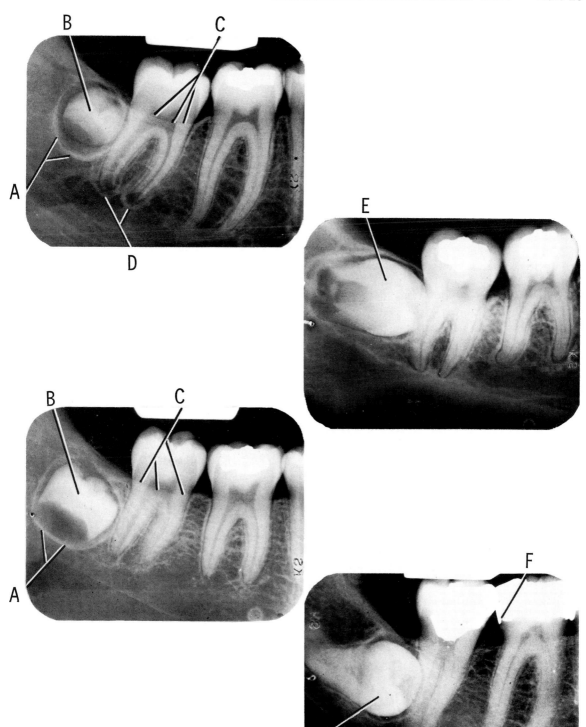

Plate 27   MANDIBULAR MOLAR REGION VIEW

A.   External oblique ridge
B.   Shadow of soft tissue
C.   Carious lesion in permanent third molar
D.   Portion of metal film holder
E.   Carious lesion in permanent second molar
F.   Normal bone trabeculation
G.   Retained root tip in soft tissue
H.   Distal surface of permanent second premolar
I.   Mandibular canal
J.   Film identification dot
K.   Radiolucent area indicating bone loss due to cariously infected tooth
L.   Lamina dura at alveolar bone crest
M.   Bone located over unerupted permanent third molar
N.   Unerupted developing permanent third molar located in developing tooth follicle
O.   Incompletely developed apices
P.   Periodontal ligament space (radiolucent line)
Q.   Cortical bone of inferior border of mandible
R.   Silver restoration
S.   Zinc phosphate cement base
T.   Gold full crown
U.   Distal root canal
V.   Interradicular bone
W.   Follicle of developing tooth
X.   Mesially impacted permanent third molar
Y.   Overlapping contacts of permanent molars
Z.   Apex of mesial root of permanent first molar

MANDIBULAR MOLAR REGION VIEW   **Plate 27**

Plate 28   MANDIBULAR MOLAR REGION VIEW

A. Distally impacted mandibular permanent third molar
B. Medullary bone resorbed indicating possible cyst formation
C. Mandibular canal
D. Cortical bone of inferior border of mandible
E. Internal oblique ridge
F. Developing crown of mandibular permanent third molar
G. Portion of metal film holder
H. Film identification dot
I. Rubber material surrounding film holder
J. Resorbed roots of mandibular permanent first molar
K. Bent corner of film

MANDIBULAR MOLAR REGION VIEW   **Plate 28**

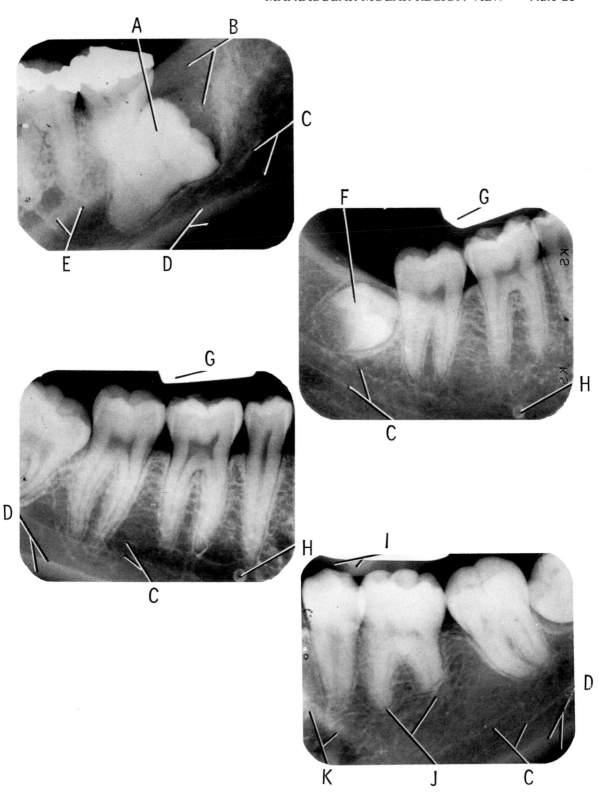

Plate 29   MANDIBULAR PREMOLAR REGION VIEW

A.   Zinc phosphate cement base
B.   Silver restoration
C.   Cast gold restoration
D.   Portion of metal film holder
E.   Rubber material surrounding film holder
F.   Cervical burnout (adumbration)
G.   Bent corner of film
H.   Mental foramen
I.   Mandibular canal
J.   Alveolar bone ridge
K.   External oblique ridge
L.   Internal oblique ridge
M.   Submandibular fossa
N.   Cast gold crown bridge abutment
O.   Cast gold bridge pontics
P.   Healed extraction sites

MANDIBULAR PREMOLAR REGION VIEW   **Plate 29**

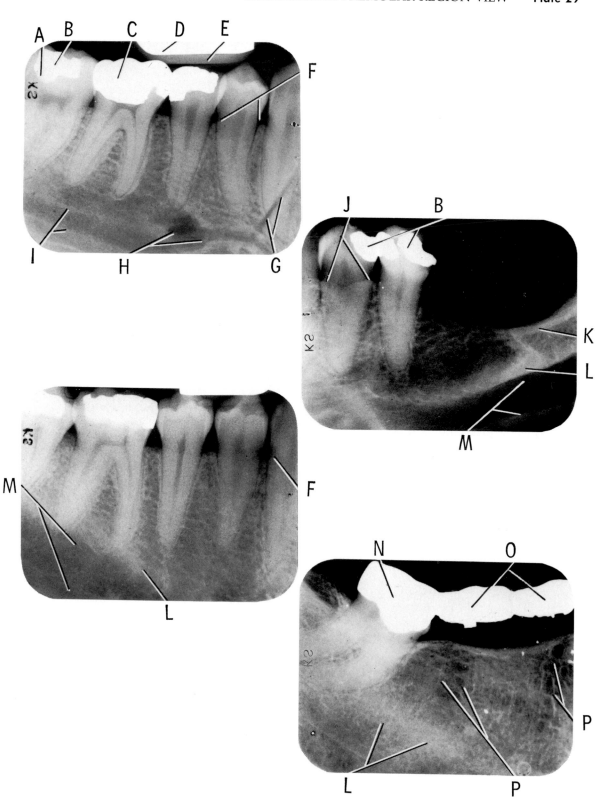

Plate 30　MANDIBULAR PREMOLAR REGION VIEW

A. Mandibular permanent canine
B. Film identification dot
C. Crown of resorbed mandibular primary first molar
D. Mandibular primary second molar
E. Erupting mandibular permanent second molar
F. Incompletely developed roots of mandibular permanent first molar
G. Developing crown of mandibular permanent second premolar
H. Developing mandibular permanent first premolar
I. Incompletely developed root of mandibular permanent first premolar
J. Lingual cusp of mandibular permanent first premolar
K. Portion of metal film holder
L. Supernumerary mandibular premolar
M. Submandibular fossa
N. Dilacerated mesial root of mandibular permanent first molar
O. Mental foramen
P. Buccal cusps of mandibular permanent first molar
Q. Unerupted mandibular permanent canine
R. Lingual cusps of mandibular permanent first molar
S. Follicle of developing permanent second molar

MANDIBULAR PREMOLAR REGION VIEW   **Plate 30**

Plate 31   MANDIBULAR PREMOLAR REGION VIEW

A. Torn film emulsion
B. Buccal cusp of mandibular permanent first premolar
C. Lingual cusp of mandibular permanent first premolar
D. Portion of metal film holder
E. Metal restorations
F. Submandibular fossa
G. Internal oblique ridge
H. Mandibular canal
I. Mental foramen
J. Sclerotic bone
K. Film identification dot
L. Shadow of portion of wooden film holder
M. Resorbed edentulous ridge
N. Bent corner of film
O. Cortical bone of inferior border of mandible
P. Bifid root of mandibular permanent second premolar
Q. Hypercementosed distal root—mandibular permanent first molar
R. Mandibular primary canine
S. Pulpally treated mandibular primary first molar
T. Chrome steel crown
U. Pulpally treated mandibular primary second molar
V. Buccal cusps of mandibular first molar
W. Partial view of unerupted mandibular permanent second molar
X. Developing mandibular second premolar
Y. Developing mandibular permanent first premolar
Z. Developing mandibular permanent canine

MANDIBULAR PREMOLAR REGION VIEW   **Plate 31**

Plate 32   MANDIBULAR PREMOLAR REGION VIEW

A.   Supernumerary teeth
B.   Nutrient foramen

MANDIBULAR PREMOLAR REGION VIEW   **Plate 32**

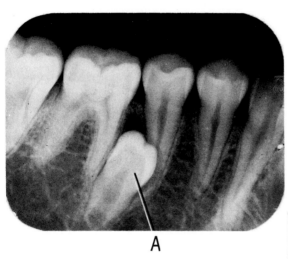

A

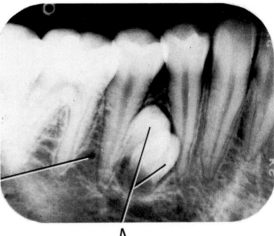

B

A

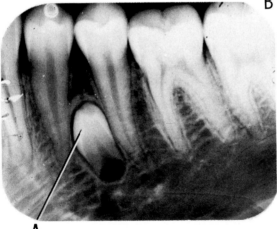

A

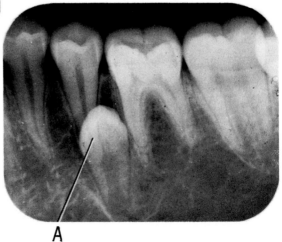

A

Plate 33   MANDIBULAR PREMOLAR–MOLAR REGION VIEW

A.   Pulp canal recession due to indirect pulp capping procedure
B.   Cervical burnout (adumbration)
C.   Mental foramen
D.   Film crease
E.   Sclerotic bone (osteosclerosis)
F.   Mandibular canal
G.   Portion of impacted mandibular permanent third molar
H.   Carious lesions
I.   Condensing osteitis
J.   Radiolucency indicating pulpal pathology, probably due to operative pulp damage
K.   Periodontal interradicular radiolucency indicating bone resorption and pathology
L.   Radiolucency around crown of erupting mandibular permanent second premolar
M.   Developing root of mandibular permanent second premolar
N.   Submandibular fossa

MANDIBULAR PREMOLAR–MOLAR REGION VIEW   **Plate 33**

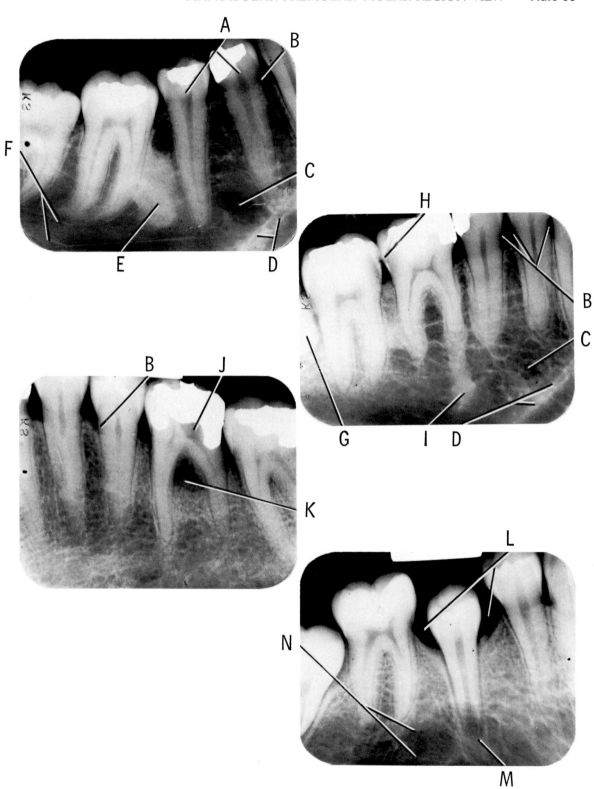

Plate 34   MANDIBULAR PREMOLAR–MOLAR REGION VIEW

A.   Internal oblique ridge
B.   External oblique ridge
C.   Film identification dot
D.   Mandibular canal
E.   Dilacerated roots
F.   Portion of metal film holder
G.   Remnant of primary second molar
H.   Area of resorbed bone over erupting permanent second molar
I.   Follicle of developing permanent second premolar
J.   Caries
K.   Submandibular fossa

MANDIBULAR PREMOLAR–MOLAR REGION VIEW   **Plate 34**

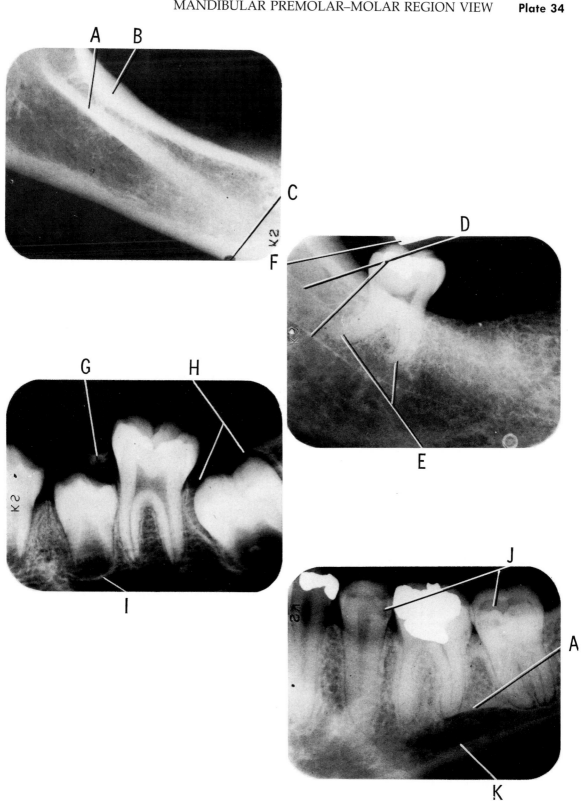

Plate 35   MANDIBULAR PREMOLAR–MOLAR REGION VIEW

A.   Submandibular fossa
B.   Ankylosed mandibular primary second molar with no developing permanent second premolar
C.   Alveolar bone level
D.   Film identification dot
E.   Lingual cusp of mandibular permanent first premolar
F.   Buccal cusp of mandibular permanent first premolar
G.   Impacted mandibular permanent second premolar
H.   Chrome steel band and loop space maintainer
I.   Metal portion of film holder
J.   Crown of developing mandibular permanent second premolar
K.   Crown of developing mandibular permanent first premolar
L.   Retained remnant of primary molar root

PART 2   *INTRAORAL RADIOGRAPHIC ANATOMY OF THE*
HUMAN MANDIBULAR ARCH
    71

MANDIBULAR PREMOLAR–MOLAR REGION VIEW   **Plate 35**

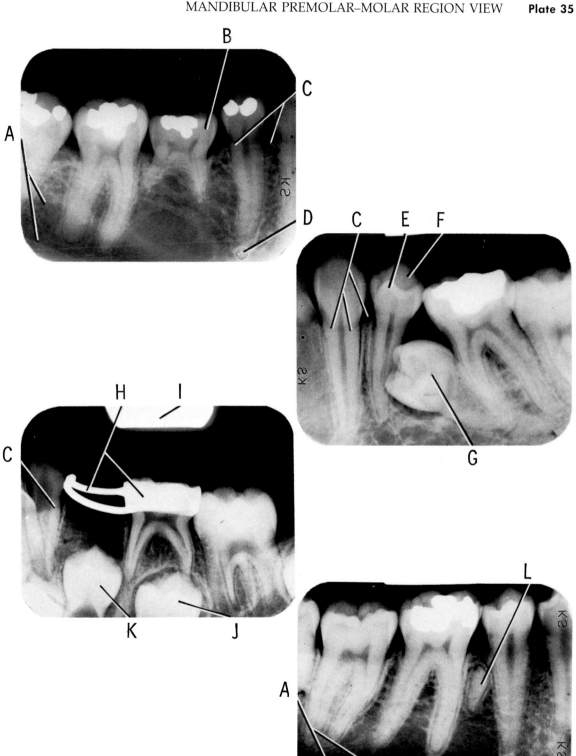

Plate 36   MANDIBULAR PREMOLAR–MOLAR REGION VIEW

A.   Film crease
B.   Mental foramen
C.   Cortical bone of inferior border of mandible
D.   Overhanging metal restorations
E.   Mandibular canal
F.   Extraction site of mandibular molar
G.   Extraction site of mandibular premolar
H.   Lamina dura
I.   Retained root tip in soft tissue
J.   Large carious lesion

MANDIBULAR PREMOLAR–MOLAR REGION VIEW   **Plate 36**

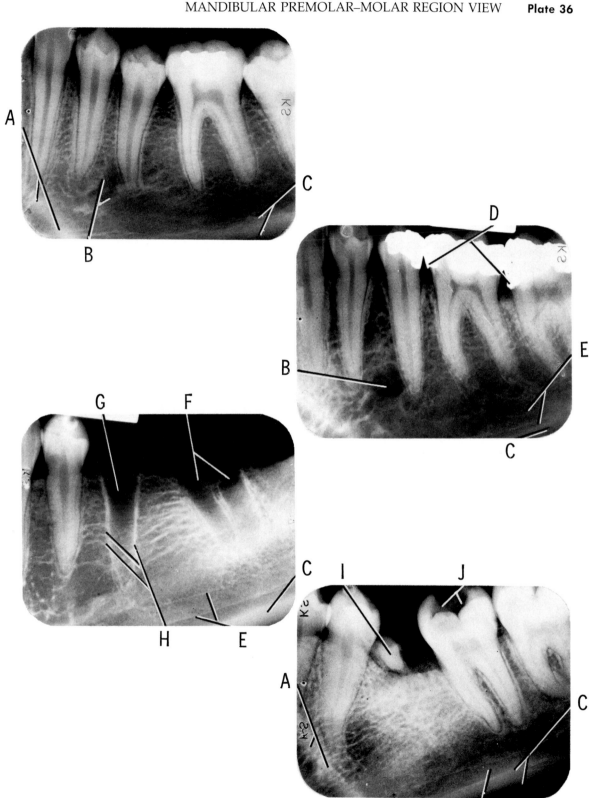

Plate 37   MANDIBULAR CANINE REGION VIEW

A.   Enamel hypoplasia
B.   Internal oblique ridge
C.   Submandibular fossa
D.   Cortical plate of inferior border of mandible
E.   Mandibular primary lateral incisor
F.   Mandibular primary canine
G.   Mandibular primary first molar
H.   Mandibular primary second molar
I.   Mandibular permanent first premolar
J.   Mandibular permanent second premolar
K.   Mandibular permanent canine
L.   Mandibular permanent lateral incisor

MANDIBULAR CANINE REGION VIEW   **Plate 37**

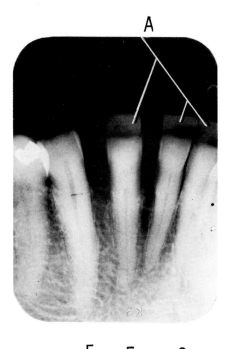

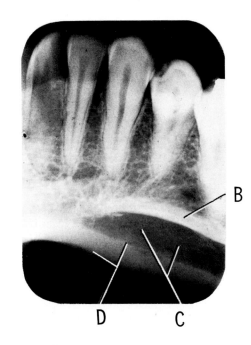

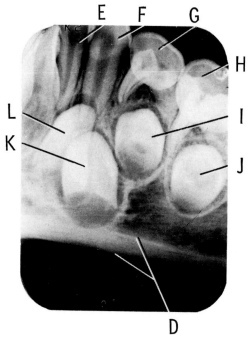

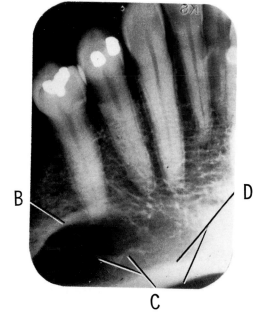

Plate 38   MANDIBULAR CANINE REGION VIEW

- **A.** Lip line
- **B.** Area of bone loss
- **C.** Alveolar bone ridge line
- **D.** Cervical abrasion
- **E.** Sclerotic bone
- **F.** Calculus
- **G.** Metal film holder
- **H.** Genial tubercle
- **I.** Lingual foramen
- **J.** Impacted mandibular permanent canine

MANDIBULAR CANINE REGION VIEW   **Plate 38**

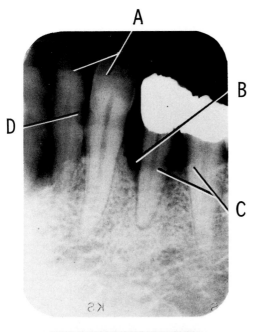

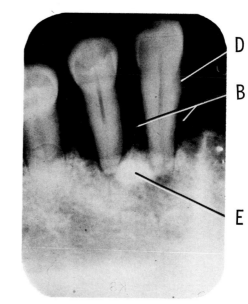

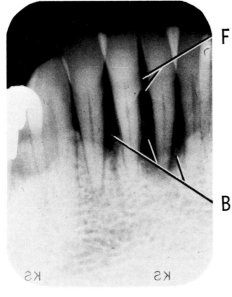

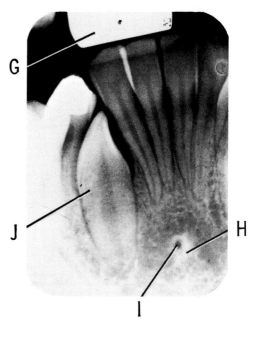

Plate 39   MANDIBULAR CANINE REGION VIEW

A.   Cervical burnout (adumbration)
B.   Shadow of alveolar bone level
C.   Calculus
D.   Area of bone resorption
E.   Developing mandibular permanent canine
F.   Exfoliating mandibular primary molar
G.   Developing root of mandibular permanent canine
H.   Cortical bone of inferior border of mandible
I.   Shadow of wooden film holder
J.   Superimposition of mandibular permanent first premolar over permanent canine

MANDIBULAR CANINE REGION VIEW   **Plate 39**

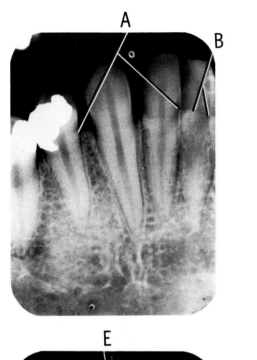

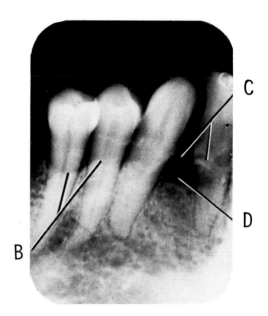

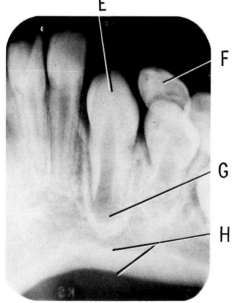

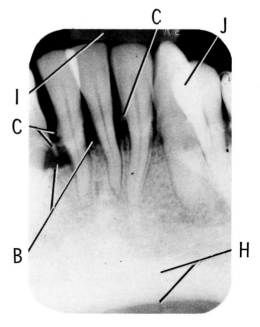

Plate 40   MANDIBULAR CANINE REGION VIEW

A.   Unerupted mandibular permanent canine in follicle
B.   Mandibular primary first molar
C.   Mandibular primary canine–root resorbed
D.   Cortical bone of inferior border of mandible
E.   Recurrent caries
F.   Periapical radiolucency due to large carious lesions
G.   Alveolar bone level
H.   Normal trabecular bone pattern
I.   Occlusal and incisal abrasion
J.   Fixer chemical stain

MANDIBULAR CANINE REGION VIEW   **Plate 40**

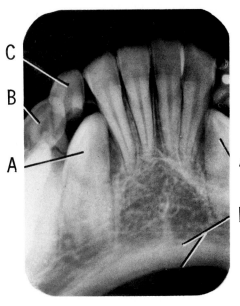

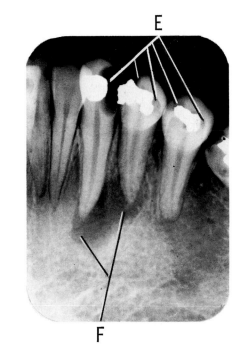

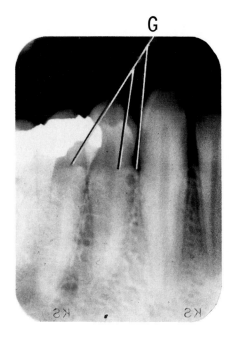

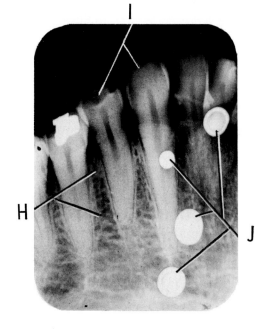

Plate 41   MANDIBULAR INCISOR REGION VIEW

A. Fractured enamel
B. Overlapped contacts
C. Abrasion
D. Level of alveolar bone
E. Lingual foramen
F. Lip line
G. Genial tubercle
H. Film crease
I. Cortical bone—inferior border of mandible
J. Narrow pulp canal (due to attrition)
K. Sclerosed pulp chamber (due to attrition)
L. Attrition
M. Mamelons
N. Film identification dot
O. Radiolucency of follicle around unerupted permanent canine

MANDIBULAR INCISOR REGION VIEW   **Plate 41**

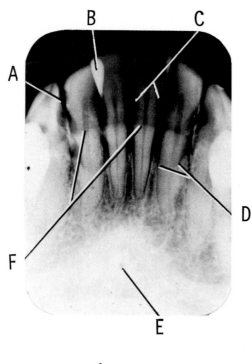

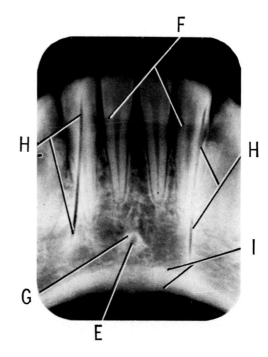

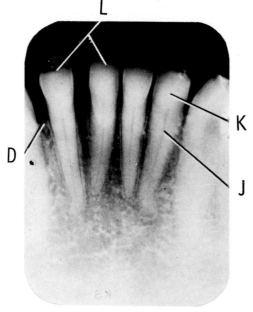

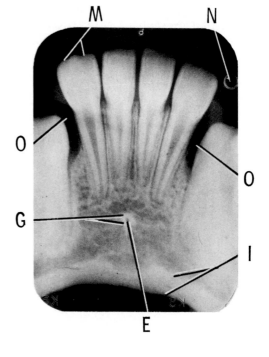

Plate 42　　MANDIBULAR INCISOR REGION VIEW

A. Radiolucent resin restorations
B. Normal thin bone
C. Genial tubercle
D. Incisal abrasion
E. Radiopaque calculus bridge
F. Alveolar ridge bone line
G. Nutrient foramen
H. Nutrient canals
I. Lip line
J. Mental ridge
K. Unerupted mandibular permanent canine
L. Cortical bone of inferior border of mandible
M. Gold crown restoration of mandibular permanent canine

MANDIBULAR INCISOR REGION VIEW   **Plate 42**

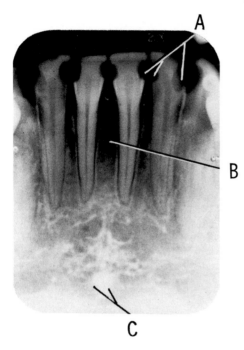

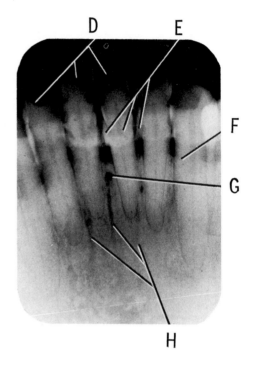

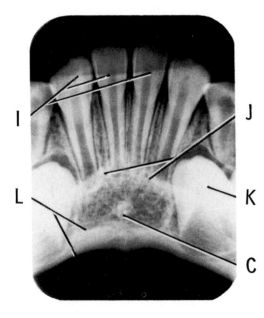

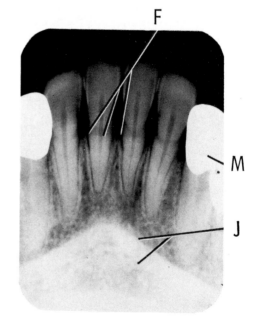

Plate 43   MANDIBULAR INCISOR REGION VIEW

A.   Permanent lateral incisor
B.   Permanent central incisor
C.   Overlapping contacts
D.   Permanent canine
E.   Genial tubercle
F.   Lingual foramen
G.   Inferior cortical plate of border of mandible
H.   Enamel
I.   Shadow of lip
J.   Calculus
K.   Alveolar bone ridge
L.   Metal film holder
M.   Rubber material surrounding film holder
N.   Film identification dot
O.   Line of fracture
P.   Metal wire used to repair fracture
Q.   Developing permanent lateral incisors in follicles
R.   Permanent central incisors with incompletely developed roots
S.   Primary lateral incisor
T.   Primary canine

MANDIBULAR INCISOR REGION VIEW   **Plate 43**

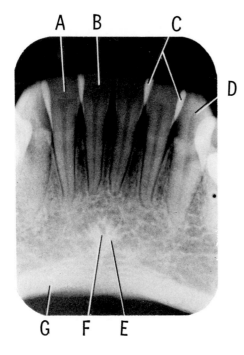

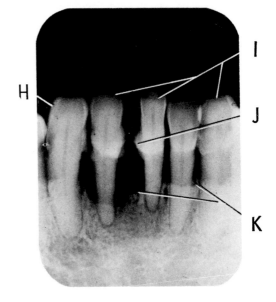

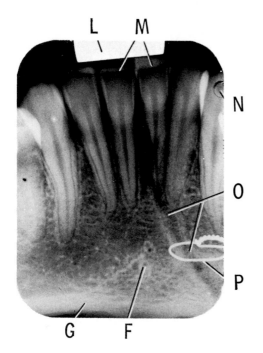

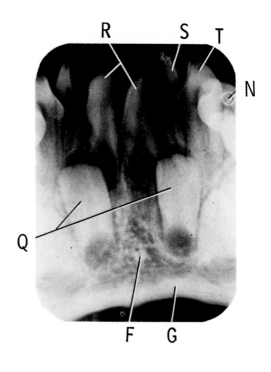

Plate 44   BITEWING VIEW OF PREMOLAR–MOLAR REGION

A.   External oblique ridge
B.   Overcontoured gold crown restoration
C.   Healed extraction site
D.   Fractured area of crown
E.   Maxillary full denture prosthetic teeth
F.   Metal pin on lingual side of prosthetic canine tooth
G.   Radiolucent space between gold restoration and tooth preparation
H.   Endodontic filling material
I.   Portion of mandibular permanent molar
J.   Pulp stones
K.   Cervical burnout (adumbration)
L.   Maxillary tuberosity

BITEWING VIEW OF PREMOLAR–MOLAR REGION   **Plate 44**

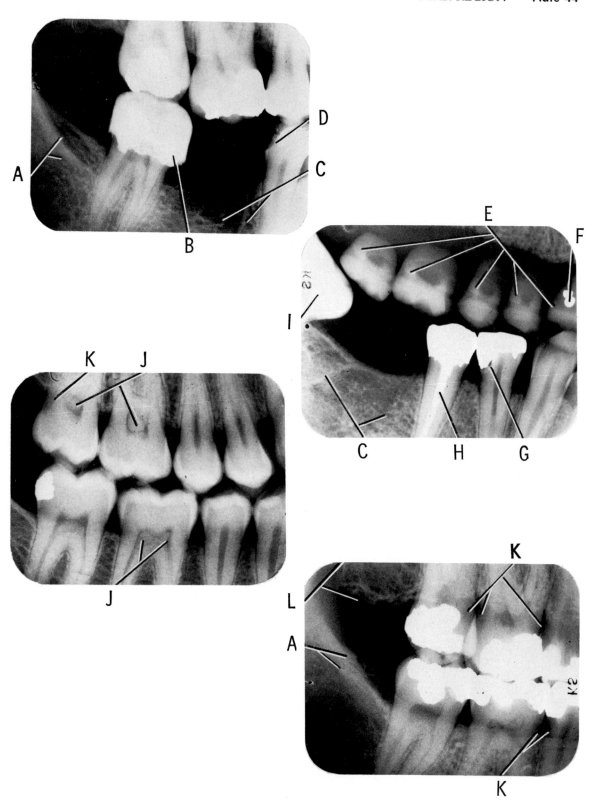

Plate 45   BITEWING VIEW OF PREMOLAR–MOLAR REGION

A.   Endodontic restoration material
B.   Overhanging restoration
C.   Gold crown restoration
D.   Bone level
E.   Metal reinforcing pins under gold crown restoration are not in pulp chamber
F.   Floor of the maxillary sinus
G.   External oblique ridge of mandible
H.   Cervical burnout (adumbration)
I.   Film identification dot
J.   Portion of unerupted mandibular permanent third molar

BITEWING VIEW OF PREMOLAR–MOLAR REGION   **Plate 45**

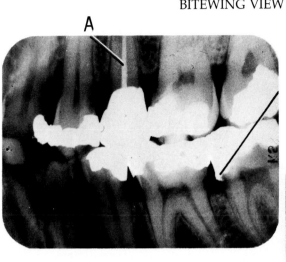

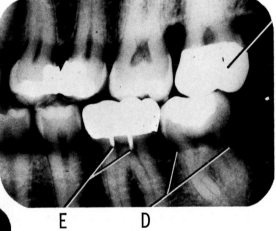

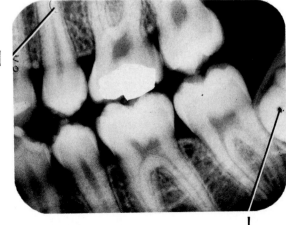

Plate 46   BITEWING VIEW OF PREMOLAR–MOLAR REGION

A.   Pulp stone
B.   Cement base under silver alloy restoration
C.   Silver alloy restoration in buccal pit
D.   Root canal
E.   Enamel
F.   Pulp chamber
G.   Carious lesion

BITEWING VIEW OF PREMOLAR–MOLAR REGION   **Plate 46**

A

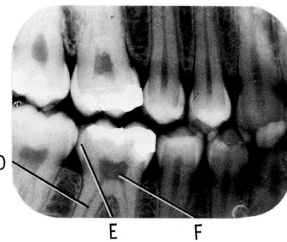

B

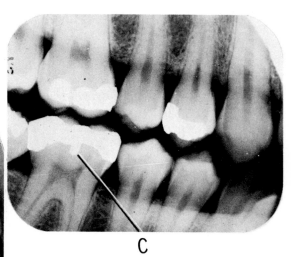

C

D

E   F

A   G

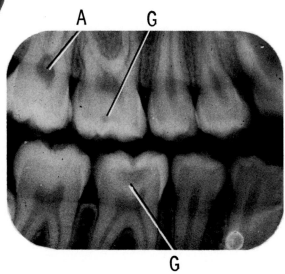

G

Plate 47   BITEWING VIEW OF PREMOLAR–MOLAR REGION

A.   Poorly contoured silver alloy restoration
B.   Carious lesion
C.   Recurrent carious lesion
D.   Pulp stone
E.   Cement base under silver alloy restoration
F.   Secondary dentin
G.   Level of alveolar bone
H.   Erupting maxillary permanent second premolar
I.   Crown remnant of maxillary primary second molar

BITEWING VIEW OF PREMOLAR–MOLAR REGION   **Plate 47**

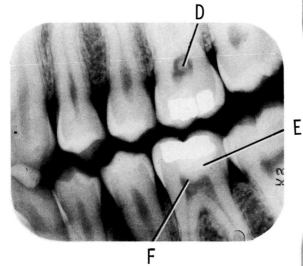

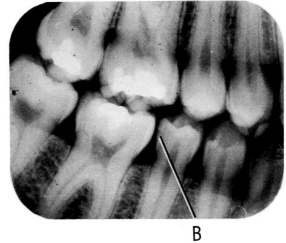

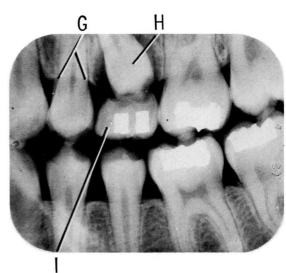

Plate 48   MAXILLARY ANTERIOR OCCLUSAL VIEW

A.   Nasal septum
B.   Nasal fossa
C.   Anterior nasal spine
D.   Nasal concha
E.   Impacted permanent central incisor
F.   Cone cut
G.   Fractured crown, permanent lateral incisor
H.   Periapical radiolucency
I.   Incisive foramen
J.   Median palatal suture
K.   Maxillary sinus
L.   Zygomatic process of maxilla

MAXILLARY ANTERIOR OCCLUSAL VIEW   **Plate 48**

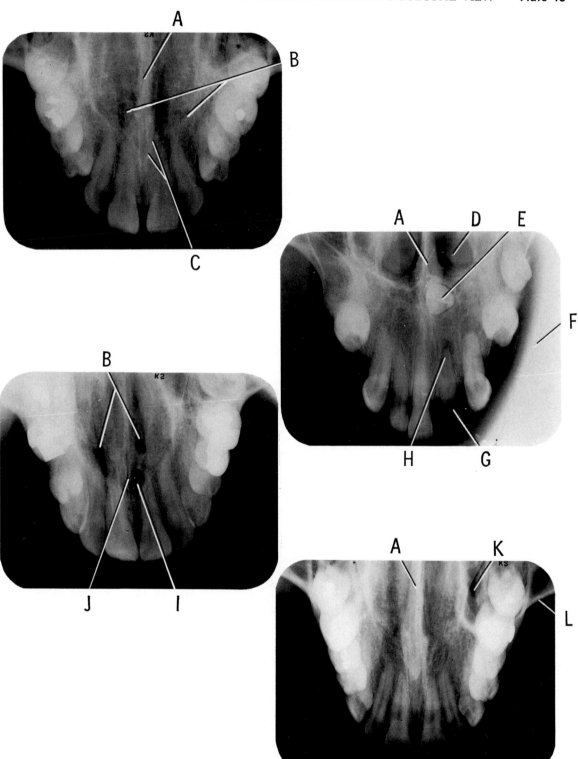

Plate 49   MAXILLARY ANTERIOR OCCLUSAL VIEW

A.   Nasal fossa
B.   Nasal septum
C.   Median palatal suture
D.   Maxillary sinus
E.   Anterior nasal spine
F.   Root canal filling
G.   Jacket crown preparation
H.   Superior foramina of incisive canal
I.   Cone cut
J.   Gold crown restorations
K.   Zygomatic process of maxilla
L.   Lateral border of nasal fossa
M.   Cartilaginous septum of nose
N.   Nasolacrimal duct
O.   Porcelain denture teeth with metal pins
P.   Retained root
Q.   Retained impacted tooth

MAXILLARY ANTERIOR OCCLUSAL VIEW   **Plate 49**

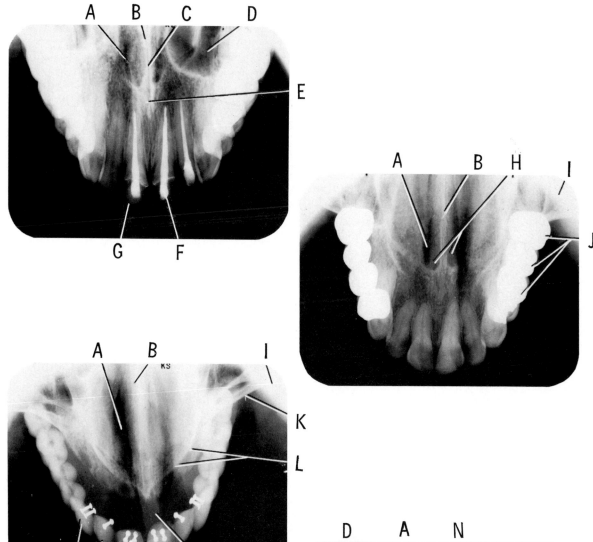

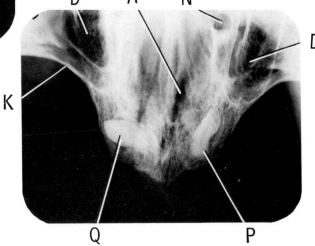

Plate 50   MANDIBULAR ANTERIOR OCCLUSAL VIEW

A.   Mental ridge
B.   Genial tubercle
C.   External oblique ridge
D.   Shadow of tongue
E.   Cone cut

MANDIBULAR ANTERIOR OCCLUSAL VIEW   **Plate 50**

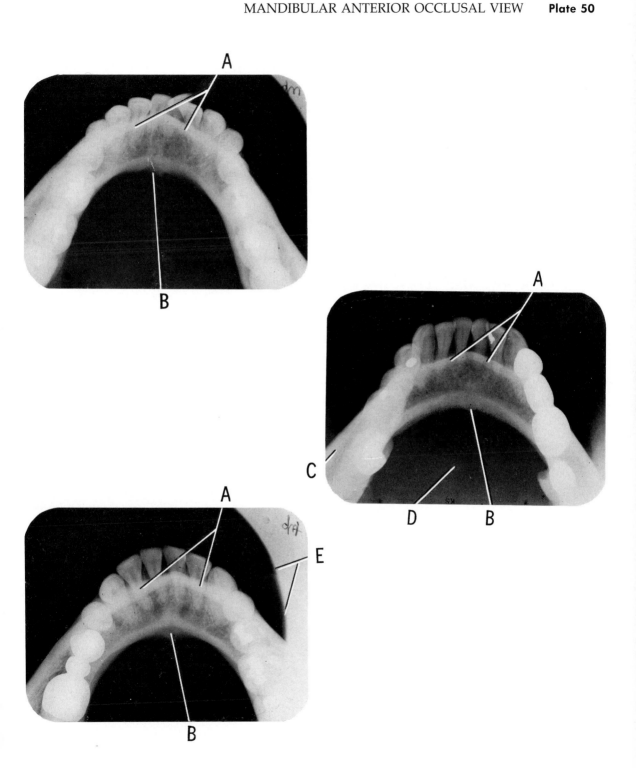

SECTION TWO

EXTRAORAL RADIOGRAPHS OF THE HUMAN SKULL

Plate 51   LATERAL OBLIQUE JAW VIEW

A. Shadow of spinal vertebrae
B. Zygomatic arch
C. Coronoid process of mandible
D. Shadow of tongue
E. Inferior border of opposite side of mandible
F. Mental foramen
G. Mandibular canal
H. Hyoid bone
I. Maxillary arch
J. Wire used to repair earlier fracture
K. Posterior wall of pharynx
L. Mandibular condyle

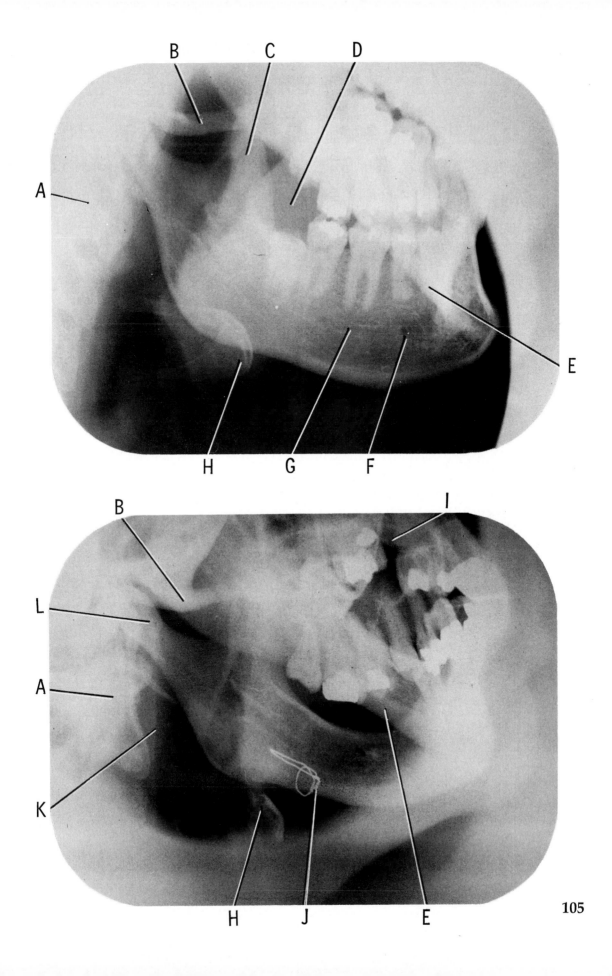

Plate 52   LATERAL OBLIQUE JAW VIEW

A.   Maxillary sinus
B.   Inferior border of opposite side of mandible
C.   Mental foramen
D.   Hyoid bone
E.   Cortical bone of inferior border of mandible
F.   Shadow of spinal vertebrae
G.   External oblique ridge
H.   Mandibular canal
I.   Mandibular foramen
J.   Sigmoid notch
K.   Coronoid process
L.   Zygomatic arch

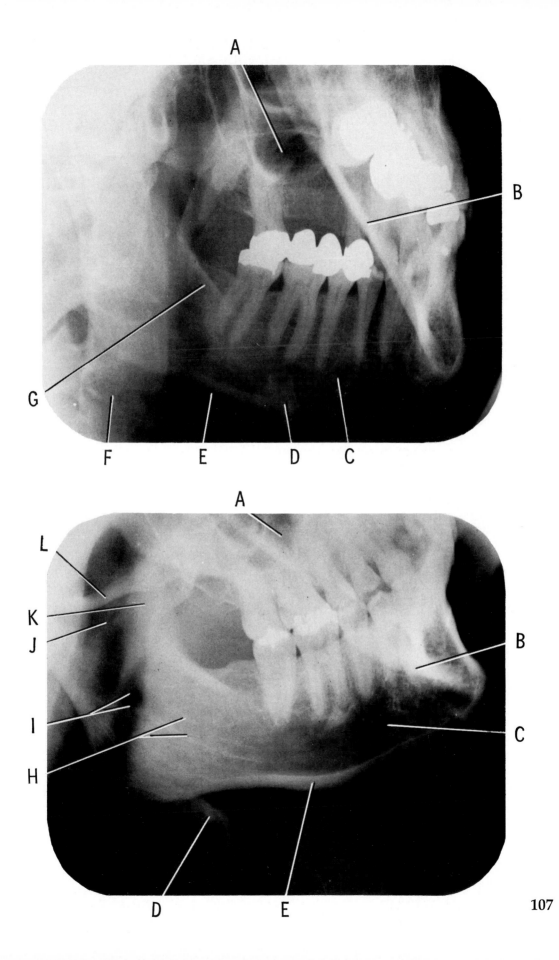

Plate 53   LATERAL OBLIQUE JAW VIEW

A.   Oropharynx
B.   Shadow of tongue
C.   Porcelain teeth of maxillary denture
D.   Mental foramen
E.   Mandibular canal
F.   Mandibular condyle
G.   Articular eminence
H.   Zygomatic arch
I.   Coronoid process of mandible
J.   Facial artery notch
K.   Styloid process

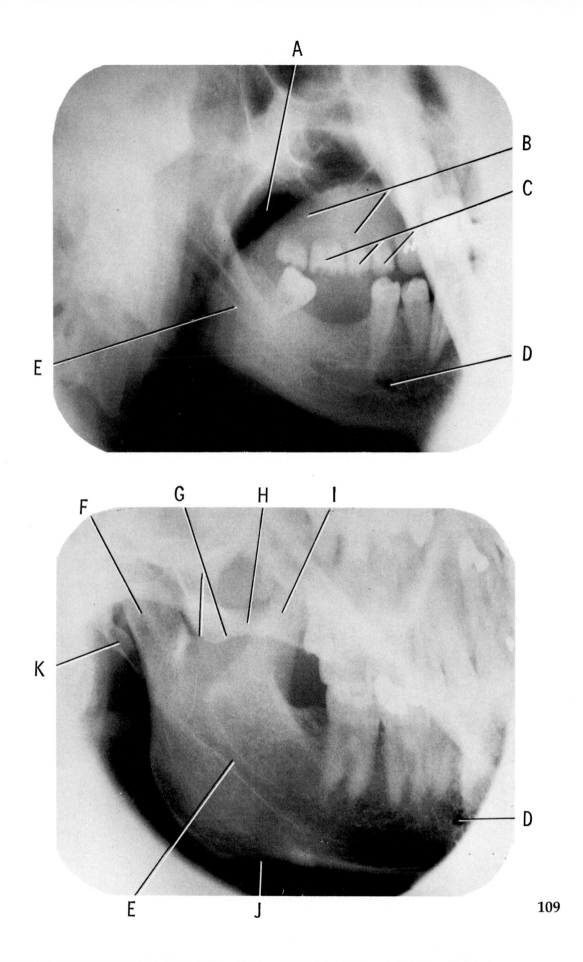

109

Plate 54   LATERAL OBLIQUE JAW VIEW

A.   Zygomatic arch
B.   Shadow of soft tissue of face
C.   Inferior border of opposite side of mandible
D.   Mental foramen
E.   Mandibular canal
F.   External oblique ridge
G.   Wall of pharynx
H.   Styloid process

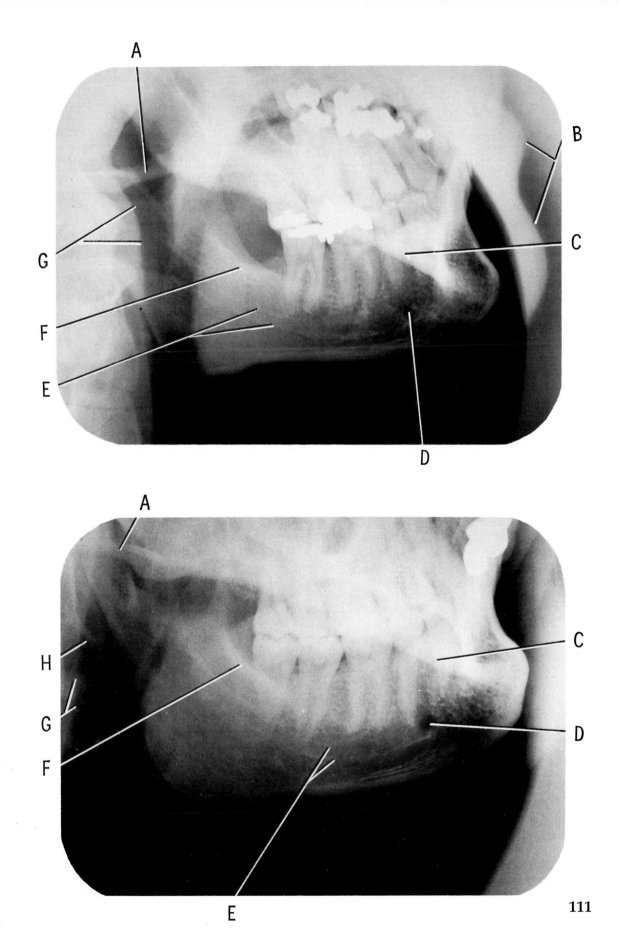

Plate 55   PANORAMIC VIEW

A. Maxillary tuberosity
B. Shadow of hard palate
C. Zygoma
D. Maxillary sinus
E. Coronoid process of mandible
F. Articular eminence
G. Glenoid fossa
H. Mandibular condyle
I. Styloid process
J. Mandibular canal
K. External oblique ridge
L. Metal bite-block
M. Shadow of tongue
N. Space between tongue and soft palate
O. Shadow of soft palate

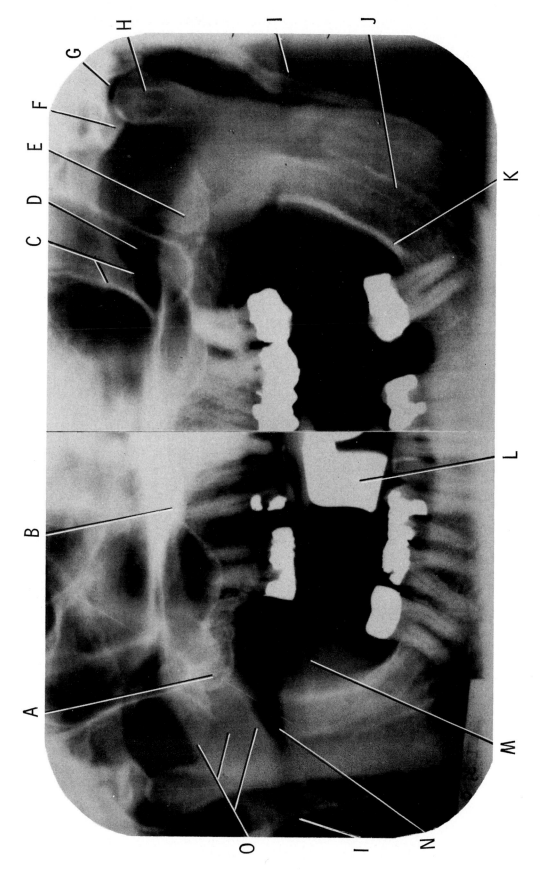

113

Plate 56   PANORAMIC VIEW (EDENTULOUS)

A. Coronoid process of mandible
B. Maxillary tuberosity
C. Nasal fossa
D. Nasal septum
E. Hard palate
F. Orbit
G. Maxillary sinus
H. Zygomatic arch
I. Articular eminence
J. Mandibular condyle
K. Cervical vertebrae
L. Facial artery notch
M. Mandibular canal
N. Plastic chin rest
O. Symphysis
P. Mental foramen
Q. Shadow of tongue
R. Angle of mandible
S. Pharynx
T. Mandibular foramen

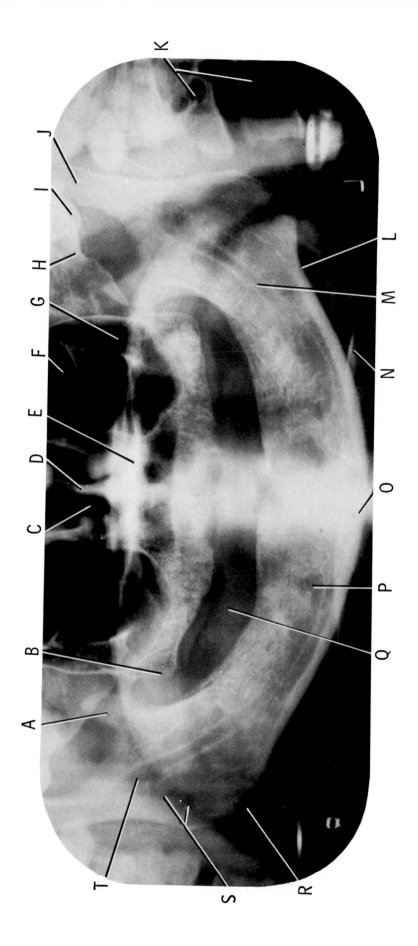

Plate 57   PANORAMIC VIEW (CHERUBISM) (FAMILIAL FIBROUS DYSPLASIA OF THE JAWS)

A. Articular eminence
B. Coronoid process of mandible
C. Nasal concha
D. Nasal septum
E. Nasal fossa
F. Maxillary sinus
G. Symphysis
H. Plastic chin rest
I. Fibro-osseous lesion
J. Angle of mandible
K. Soft tissue of external ear (lobule)
L. Cervical vertebra
M. Mandibular condyle
N. External auditory meatus
O. Glenoid fossa

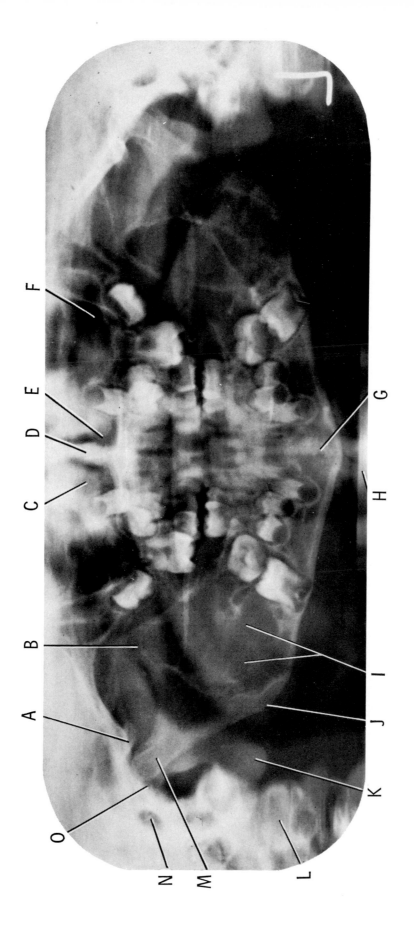

Plate 58   PANORAMIC VIEW

Film damaged by static electricity

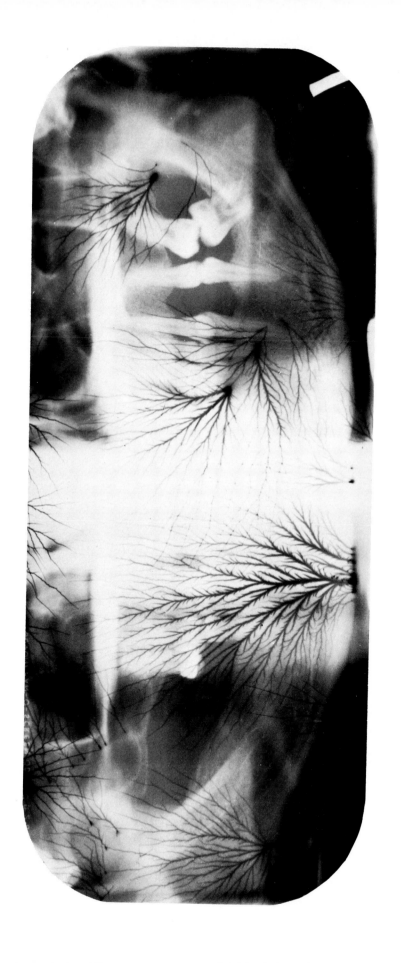

119

Plate 59   PANORAMIC VIEW

A. Nasal fossa
B. Nasal septum
C. Hard palate
D. Maxillary sinus
E. Zygomatic arch
F. Articular eminence
G. Glenoid fossa
H. Mandibular condyle
I. Mental foramen
J. Symphysis
K. Mandibular canal
L. Cervical vertebra
M. Mandibular foramen
N. Styloid process

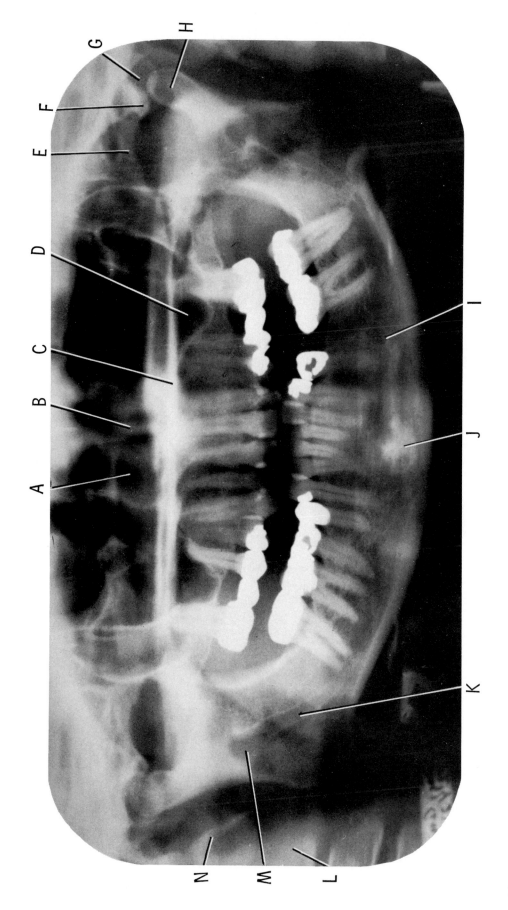

Plate 60   PANORAMIC VIEW

A. Maxillary sinus
B. Nasal fossa
C. Hard palate
D. Zygomatic arch
E. Mandibular canal
F. Oropharynx
G. Symphysis
H. External oblique ridge
I. Soft palate

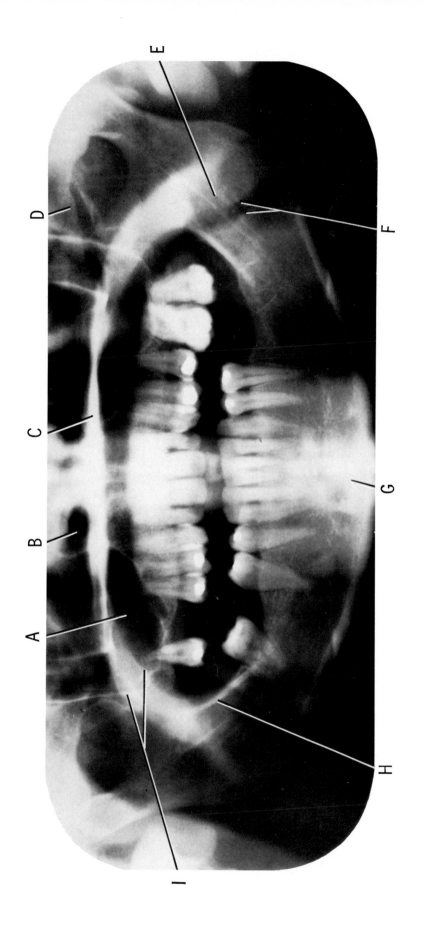

Plate 61   PANORAMIC VIEW (EDENTULOUS)

A. Mandibular notch
B. Nasal concha
C. Nasal septum
D. Nasal fossa
E. Hard palate
F. Articular eminence
G. Glenoid fossa
H. Mandibular condyle
I. External oblique ridge
J. Mental foramen
K. Shadow of ramus of opposite side

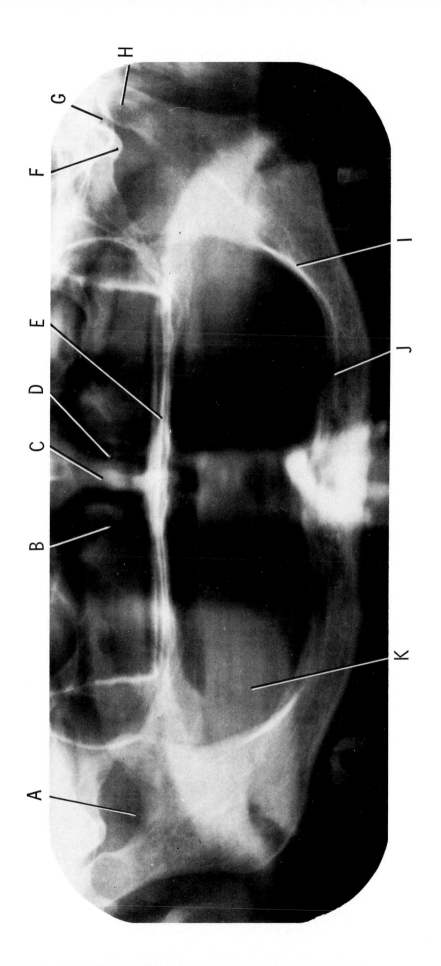

125

Plate 62   PANORAMIC VIEW

A. Maxillary sinus
B. Area of no radiation exposure
C. Nasal septum
D. Nasal fossa and concha
E. Hard palate
F. Plastic chin rest
G. Large carious lesion
H. Maxillary permanent lateral incisor
I. Maxillary permanent central incisor of opposite side
J. Carious lesion
K. Shadow of plastic chin rest of opposite side
L. Shadow of ramus of opposite side
M. Soft tissue of external ear (lobule)
N. External auditory meatus

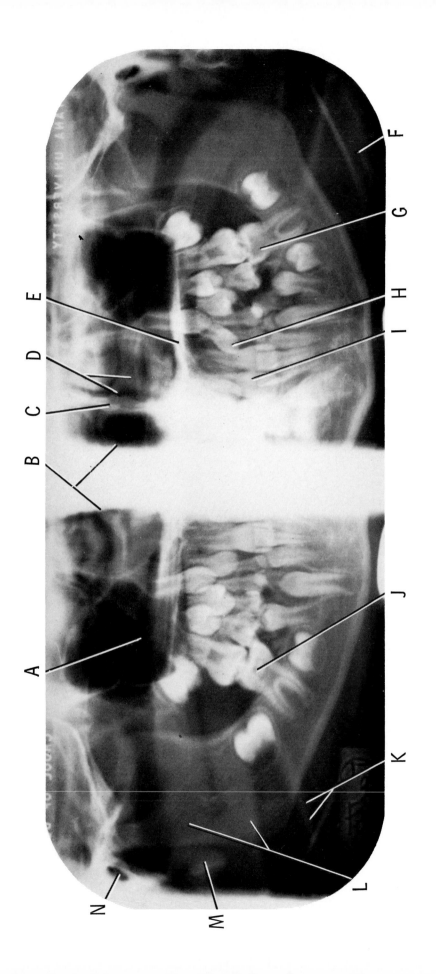

127

Plate 63   LATERAL HEADPLATE VIEW

A. External cortical plate
B. Internal cortical plate
C. Coronal suture
D. Artifact
E. Anterior clinoid process
F. Roof of orbit
G. Nasal fossa
H. Nasal bone
I. Anterior nasal spine
J. Developing mandibular permanent second molar in follicle
K. Sphenoid sinus
L. External auditory meatus
M. Pituitary fossa in sella turcica
N. Mastoid process
O. Occipitomastoid suture
P. Posterior clinoid process
Q. Lambdoid suture
R. Squamous suture

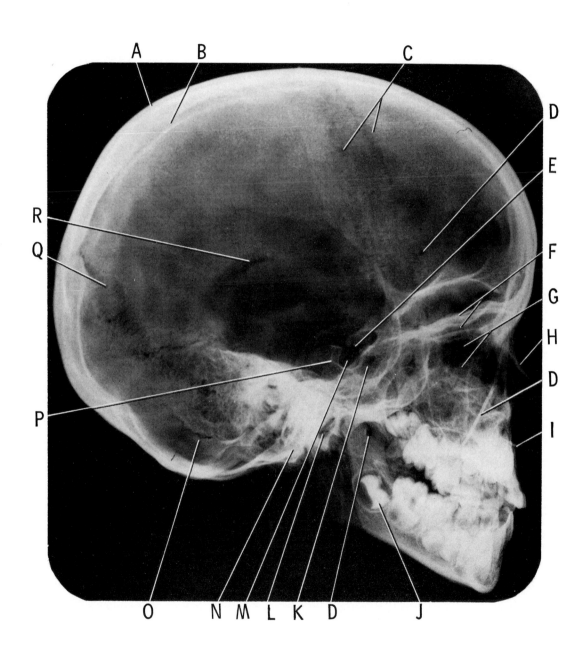

Plate 64   LATERAL HEADPLATE VIEW

A. Metal ear rod
B. Pituitary fossa in sella turcica
C. Roof of orbit
D. Anterior clinoid process
E. Frontal sinus
F. Plastic orbital pointer
G. Posterior clinoid process
H. Sphenoid sinus
I. Orbit
J. Nasal fossa
K. Anterior nasal spine
L. Floor of nasal fossa
M. Roof of maxillary sinus
N. Maxillary sinus

O. Posterior border of tongue
P. Oropharynx
Q. Hyoid bone
R. Posterior pharyngeal wall
S. Body of third cervical vertebra
T. Body of fourth cervical vertebra
U. Body of fifth cervical vertebra
V. Body of axis
W. Spinous processes of third, fourth and fifth cervical vertebrae
X. Soft palate
Y. Spinous process of axis
Z. Spinous process of atlas

a. Nasopharynx
b. Odontoid process of axis
c. Anterior tubercle of atlas
d. Occipital eminence

e. Occipital condyle
f. Mastoid air cells
g. Shadow of petrosal pyramid of temporal bone

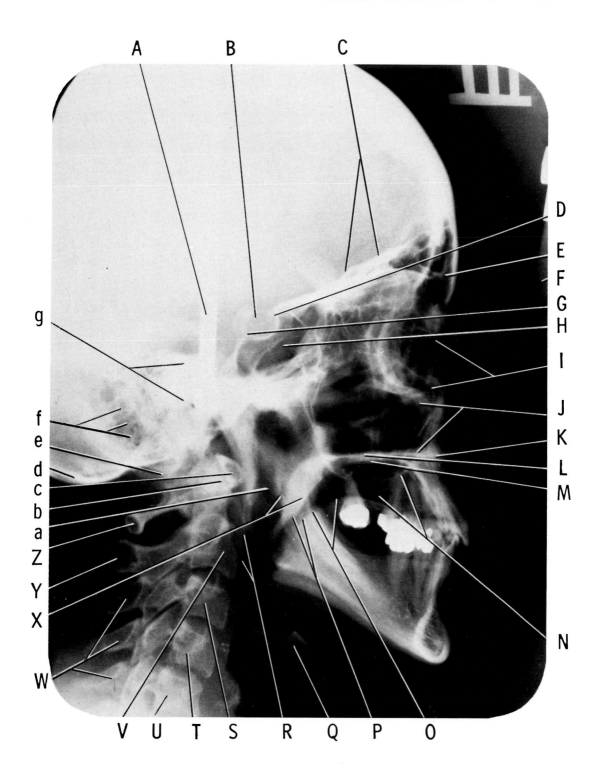

Plate 65   LATERAL HEADPLATE VIEW

A.	Coronal suture
B.	Inner cortical plate
C.	Outer cortical plate
D.	Roof of orbit
E.	Frontal sinus
F.	Orbit
G.	Sphenoid sinus
H.	Maxillary sinus superimposed over nasal fossa
I.	Radiopaque material painted on the dorsum of the tongue
J.	Lip of maxilla
K.	Lip of mandible
L.	Mandibular permanent first and second premolars

M.	Mandibular permanent first and second molars
N.	Unerupted mandibular permanent third molar
O.	Soft palate
P.	Hyoid bone
Q.	Oropharynx
R.	Nasopharynx
S.	Fourth cervical vertebra
T.	Third cervical vertebra
U.	Axis
V.	Atlas
W.	Pituitary fossa in sella turcica
X.	Mastoid air cells
Y.	Plastic ear rod and head holder
Z.	Posterior clinoid process

a.   Metal hairpins

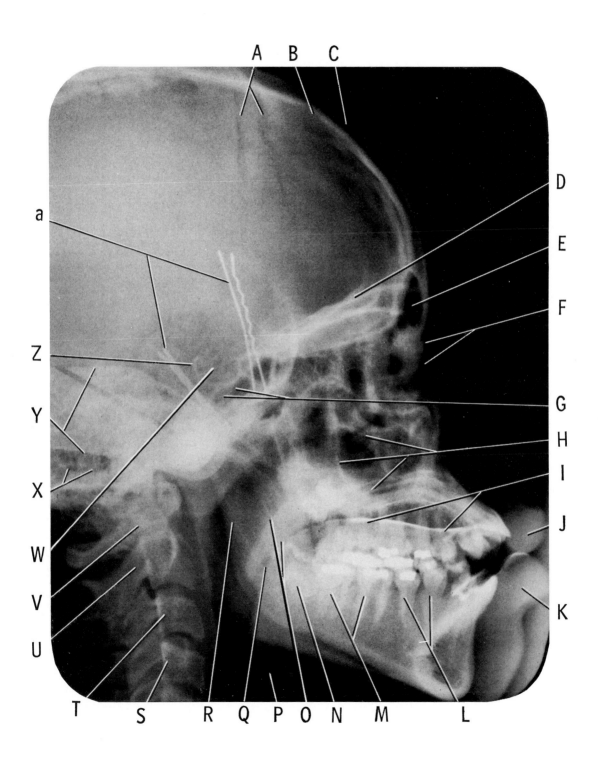

Plate 66   LATERAL HEADPLATE VIEW

A.	Patient identification plate	**N.**	Maxillary permanent first premolar
B.	Inner cortical plate	**O.**	Maxillary permanent second premolar
C.	Outer cortical plate	**P.**	Maxillary permanent first molar
D.	Posterior clinoid process	**Q.**	Maxillary primary molars
E.	Pituitary fossa in sella turcica	**R.**	Mandibular permanent first premolar
F.	Roof of orbit	**S.**	Mandibular primary second molar
G.	Anterior clinoid process	**T.**	Mandibular permanent second premolar
H.	Frontal sinus		
I.	Sphenoid sinus	**U.**	Mandibular permanent first molar
J.	Orbit	**V.**	Maxillary permanent second molar
K.	Maxillary sinus superimposed over nasal fossa	**W.**	Mandibular permanent second molar
		X.	Hyoid bone
L.	Hard palate	**Y.**	Oropharynx
M.	Unerupted maxillary permanent canine	**Z.**	Soft palate

---

a.	Nasopharynx	**g.**	Odontoid process of axis
b.	Pharyngeal wall	**h.**	Mastoid air cells
c.	Fourth cervical vertebra	**i.**	Outer cortical plate of occipital bone
d.	Third cervical vertebra	**j.**	Inner cortical plate of occipital bone
e.	Axis	**k.**	Plastic ear rod and head holder
f.	Atlas	**l.**	Lambdoid suture

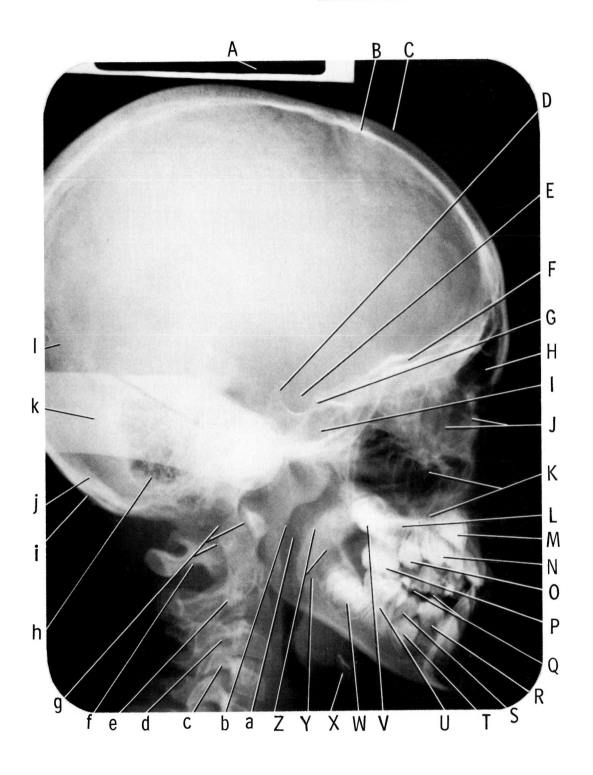

Plate 67   POSTEROANTERIOR HEADPLATE VIEW

A. Sagittal suture
B. Coronal suture
C. Greater wing of sphenoid
D. Superior border of orbit
E. Nasal septum
F. Nasal concha
G. Primary central incisor of maxilla
H. Unerupted permanent first molar of mandible
I. Angle of mandible
J. Inferior border of mandible
K. Shadow of cervical vertebrae
L. Primary cuspid of mandible
M. Unerupted mandibular permanent central incisor
N. Unerupted mandibular permanent lateral incisor
O. Unerupted mandibular permanent canine
P. Mandibular primary left central incisor
Q. Mandibular primary right central incisor
R. Unerupted maxillary permanent central incisor
S. Unerupted maxillary permanent first molar
T. Maxillary sinus
U. Foramen rotundum
V. Crista galli

POSTEROANTERIOR HEADPLATE VIEW   **Plate 67**

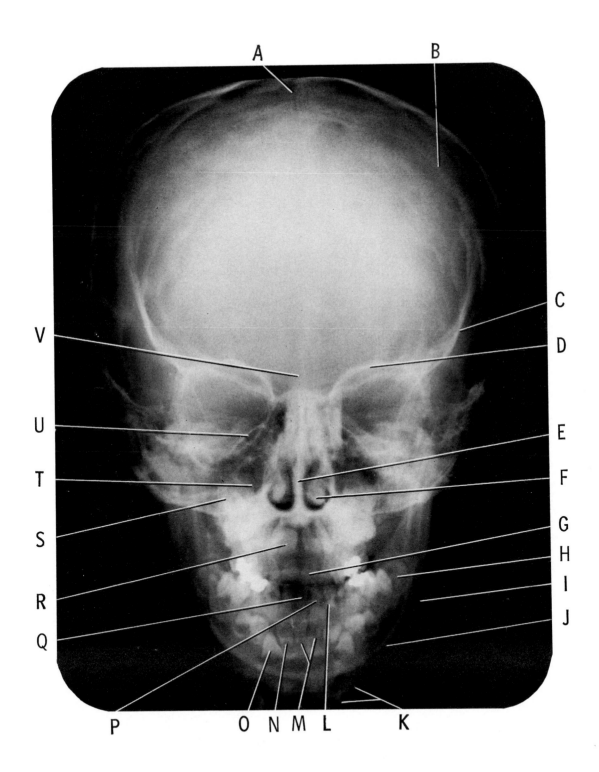

Plate 68 POSTEROANTERIOR HEADPLATE VIEW

A. Midsagittal suture
B. Frontal sinus
C. Plastic head positioner
D. Mastoid air cells
E. Nasal septum
F. Nasal concha (turbinate)
G. Anterior nasal spine
H. Unerupted maxillary permanent second molar
I. Unerupted mandibular permanent second molar
J. Maxillary permanent central incisors
K. Mandibular permanent central incisors
L. Mandibular permanent lateral incisor
M. Unerupted mandibular permanent canine
N. Mandibular permanent first premolar
O. Angle of mandible
P. Neck of ramus of mandible
Q. Maxillary sinus
R. Petrous portion of temporal bone
S. Orbit

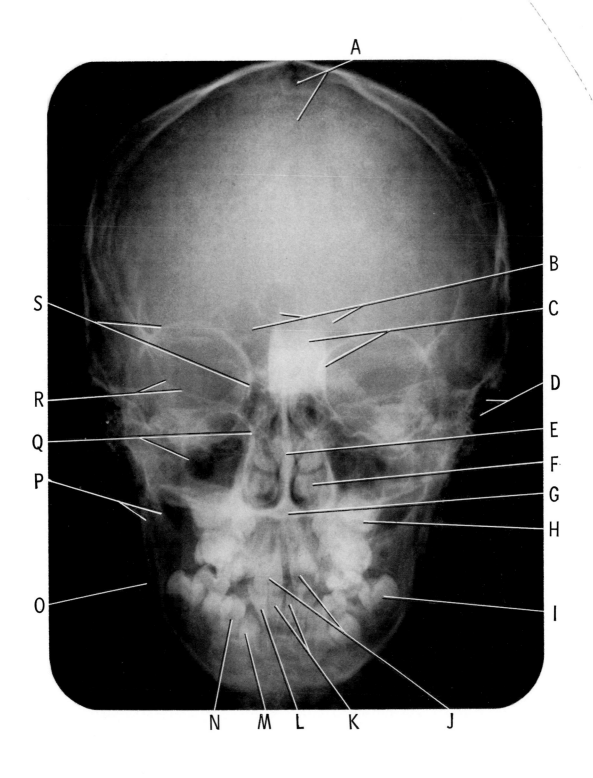

ιTERS' SINUS HEADPLATE VIEW

A.   Frontal sinus
B.   Orbit
C.   Nasal septum
D.   Nasal conchae
E.   Maxillary sinus
F.   Zygomatic arch
G.   Anterior teeth of mandible
H.   Odontoid process of axis
I.   Foramen magnum
J.   Inferior border of mandible
K.   Posterior border of ramus of mandible
L.   Foramen rotundum

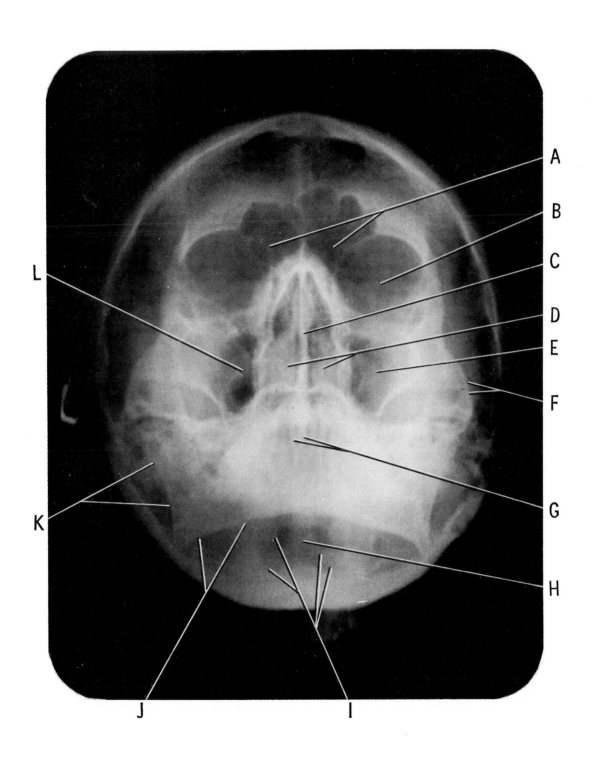

Plate 70   TEMPOROMANDIBULAR JOINT VIEW (UPDEGRAVE)

A. Open position
B. Rest position
C. Closed position
D. Glenoid fossa
E. Cranium interior
F. Head of mandibular condyle
G. Articular eminence
H. External auditory meatus

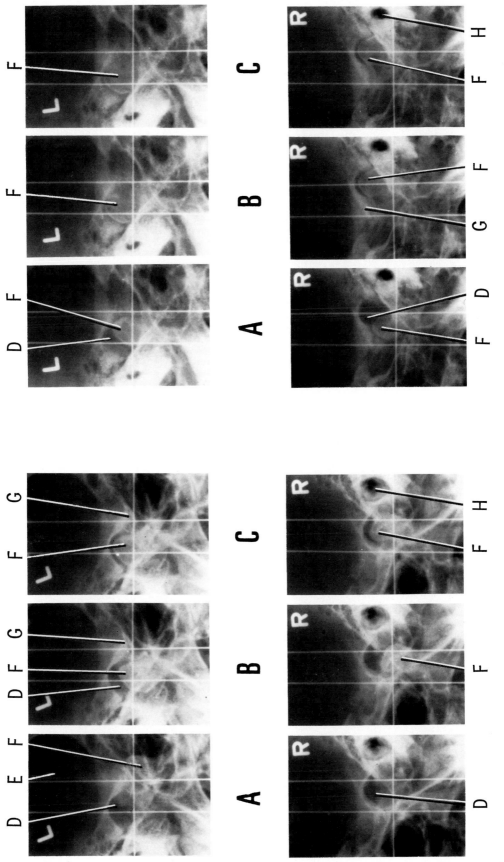

Plate 71   TEMPOROMANDIBULAR JOINT VIEW (TRANSORBITAL)

A.   Zygomatic arch
B.   Medial third of head of condyle
C.   Lateral third of head of condyle
D.   Neck of condyle
E.   Styloid process
F.   Mastoid process

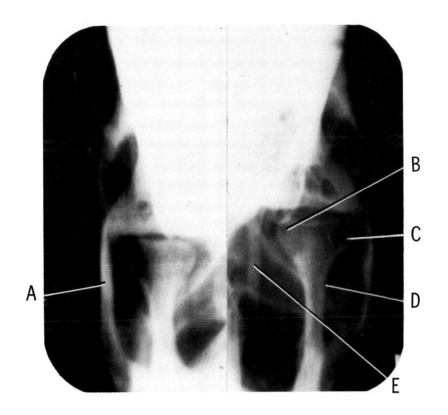

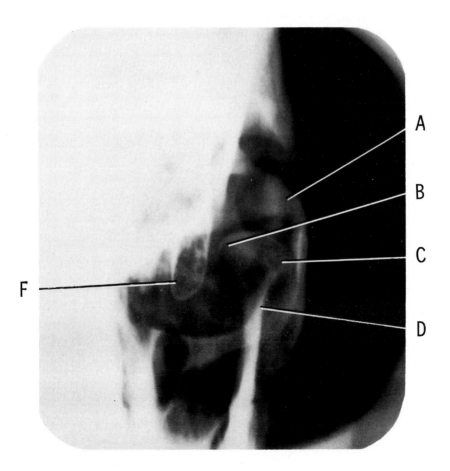

Plate 72   TEMPOROMANDIBULAR JOINT VIEW

A.   The single arrowhead indicates an area of agenesis of the mandibular condyle. The double arrows indicate a normal mandibular condyle on the opposite side.

B.   This is a transpharyngeal view of the mandibular condyle. The single arrow indicates the location of the condyle; the arrowhead points to the sella turcica. The radiolucency inferior and anterior to the sella is the sphenoid sinus.

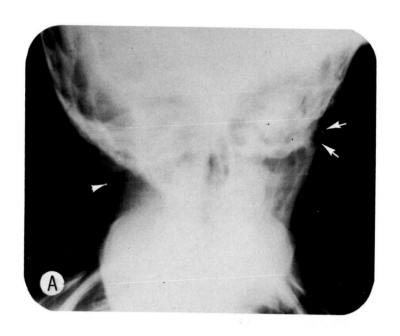

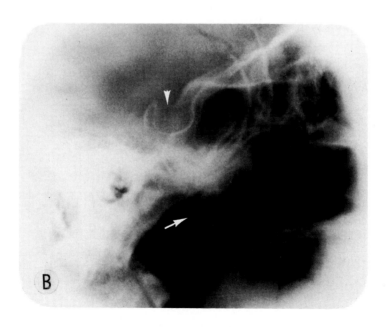

Plate 73   TEMPOROMANDIBULAR JOINT VIEW

A.   This is a straight lateral tomogram of the right condyle of a 26-year-old patient.
B.   This is a corrected axis tomogram of the same condyle. It displays a more accurate radiographic view of this condyle.
(Tomograms courtesy of Dr. A. Sondhi.)

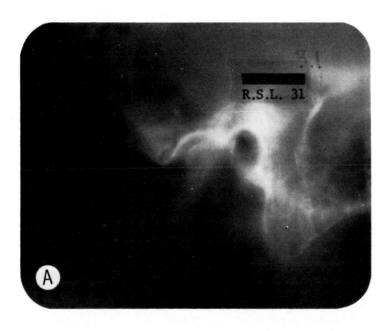

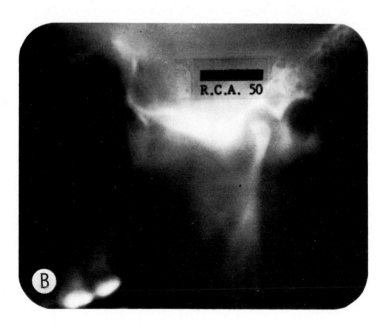

Plate 74   TEMPOROMANDIBULAR JOINT VIEW

A.   This right corrected axis tomogram reveals a flat condyle (arrowheads). There
           was pain in the temporomandibular joint.
B.   This is a right corrected axis tomogram showing a cystic erosive change (arrow)
           in the condyle. The patient was a 50-year-old woman with a history of dull
           pain in the temporomandibular joint.
           (Tomograms courtesy of Dr. A. Sondhi.)

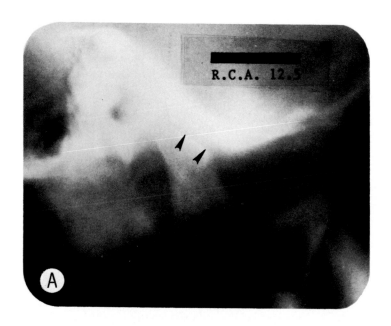

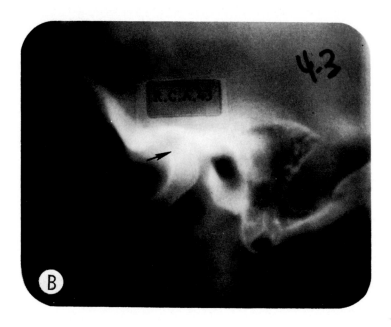

Plate 75   TEMPOROMANDIBULAR JOINT VIEW

A.   The condyle shown here was fixed in a dislocated position (not in the glenoid fossa) following a subcondylar osteotomy. The fossa had calcified during the ensuing years (arrowheads), and although the patient had achieved some accommodation to this condition, there was persistent temporomandibular joint pain as well.

B.   In this case, diagnosed as degenerative osteoarthritic change and loss of joint space (in a 49-year-old woman who experienced pain in the temporomandibular joint), there is a bone spur on the condyle (arrow). The external auditory meatus (1) and the mastoid air cells (2) are identified.
(Tomograms courtesy of Dr. A. Sondhi.)

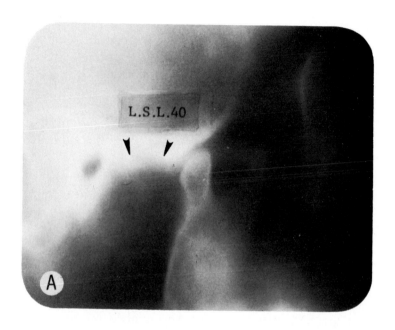

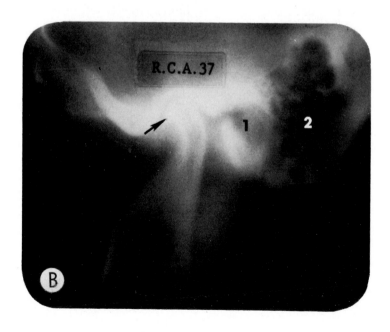

Plate 76   TEMPOROMANDIBULAR JOINT VIEW

A.   Corrected axis radiograph showing left condyle position (arrowhead) at physiologic rest.

B.   Corrected axis radiograph showing left condyle position (arrowhead) with maximum intercuspation.

C.   Corrected axis radiograph showing limited translation of left condyle (arrowhead) with maximum opening.
      (Radiographs courtesy of Dr. J. Green.)

TEMPOROMANDIBULAR JOINT VIEW   **Plate 76**

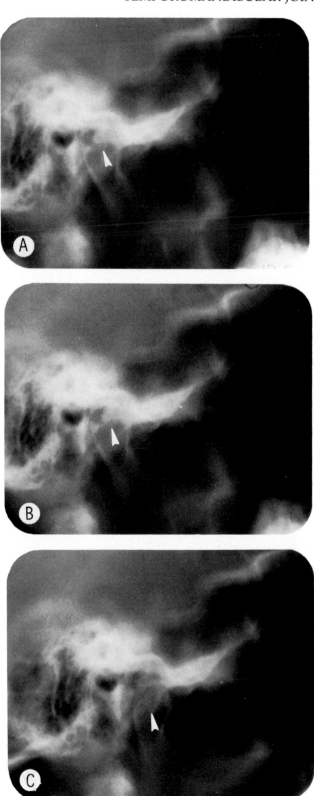

Plate 77   TEMPOROMANDIBULAR JOINT VIEW

A, B, C.   Corrected axis tomograms showing decreased joint space and posterior positioning of left condyle (arrowheads) due to anteriorly displaced meniscus. (Tomograms courtesy of Dr. J. Green.)

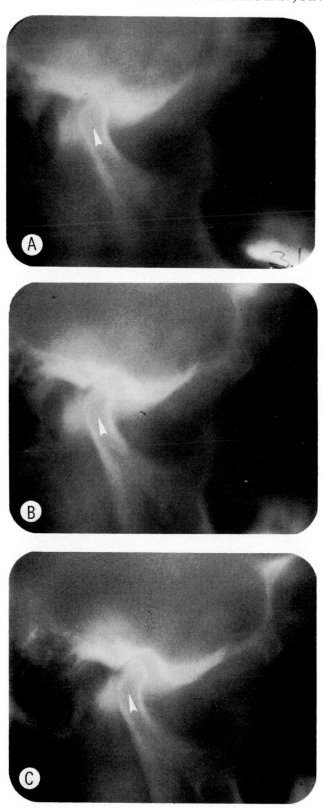

Plate 78   TEMPOROMANDIBULAR JOINT VIEW

A.   Corrected axis radiograph showing right condyle position at physiologic rest (osteophytic spur [arrowhead] visible on anterior surface of condyle).

B.   Corrected axis radiograph showing right condyle position at maximum inter-cuspation (osteophytic spur [arrowhead] visible on anterior surface of condyle).

C.   Corrected axis radiograph showing limited translation of right condyle with maximum opening (osteophytic spur [arrowhead] visible on anterior surface of condyle).

(Radiographs courtesy of Dr. J. Green.)

TEMPOROMANDIBULAR JOINT VIEW   **Plate 78**

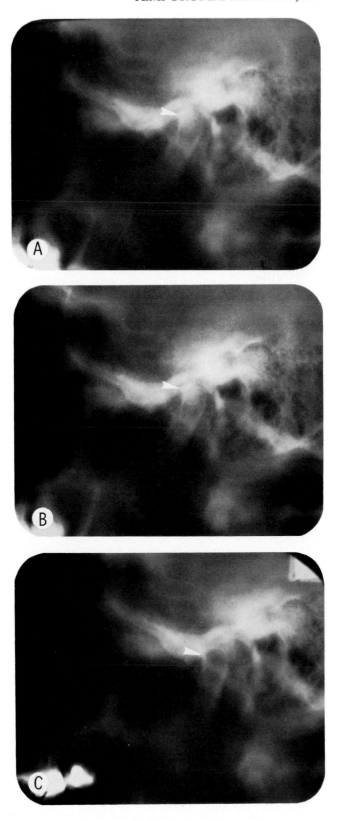

Plate 79   TEMPOROMANDIBULAR JOINT VIEW

A, B.   Corrected axis tomograms showing osteophytic spur (arrowheads) on right condyle, indicating degenerative joint disease (osteoarthritis).
(Tomograms courtesy of Dr. J. Green.)

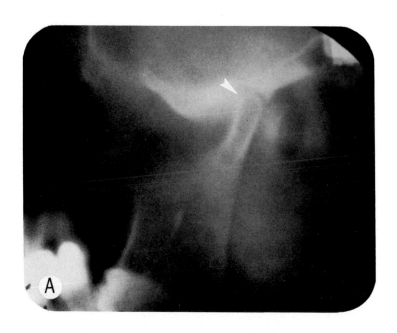

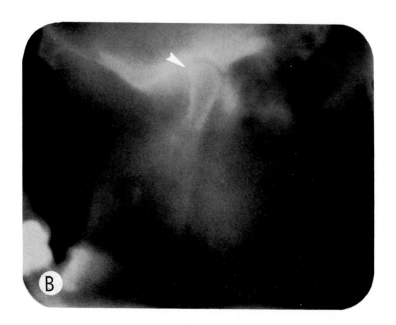

SECTION THREE

FILM ARTIFACTS AND TECHNICAL ERRORS

Plate 80   FILM OVERLAPPING DURING DEVELOPMENT

During film development a second film overlapped these films, leaving an artifact over these crowns (black arrowheads).

FILM OVERLAPPING DURING DEVELOPMENT   **Plate 80**

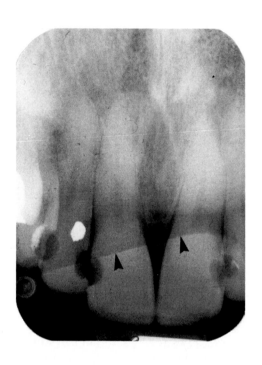

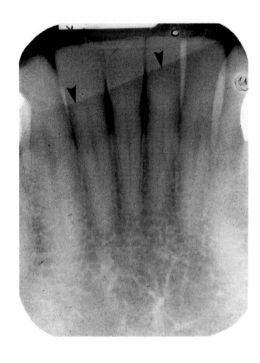

Plate 81   STATIC ELECTRICITY ARTIFACTS

The radiolucent jagged lines seen on the molar crowns are the result of static electricity. This result sometimes occurs during the opening of film packets in the darkroom.

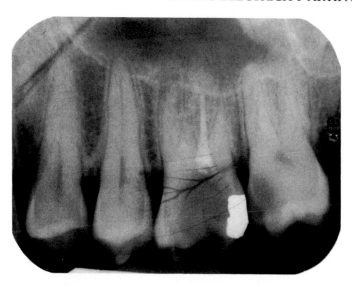

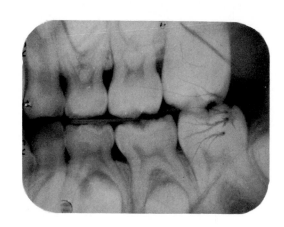

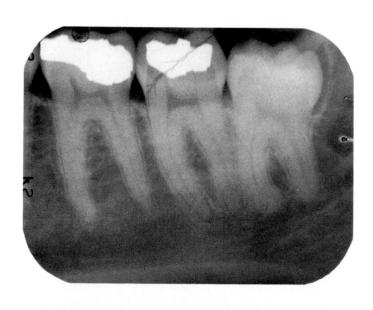

Plate 82 LEAD APRON COLLAR ARTIFACTS

The large radiopaque area superimposed over the lower half of these radiographs is the outline of the lead apron collar. Note the radiolucent spots lined up in a row. They indicate where the thyroid protective collar is sewn to the lead protective apron.

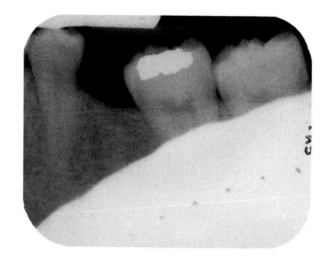

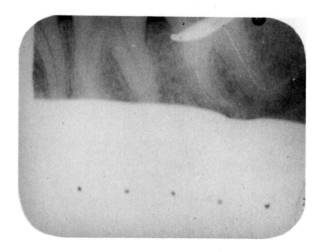

Plate 83   LEAD BACKING ARTIFACTS

When placed in the patient's mouth, the film packet sometimes gets folded over itself. The lead backing in the film packet appears superimposed over the roots of the teeth in **B.** Lead backing artifacts are also seen in **A** and **C.**

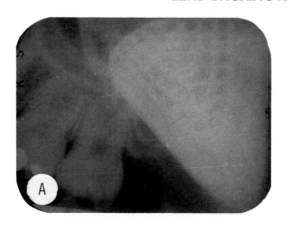

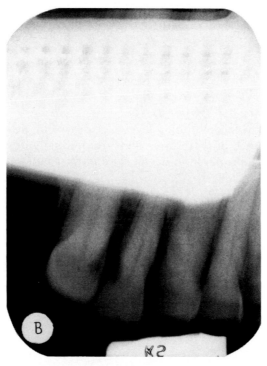

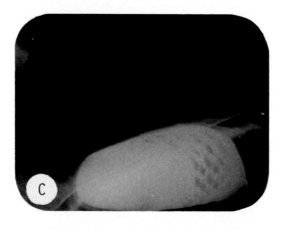

Plate 84   DEVELOPER SOLUTION LEVEL ARTIFACTS

Because the developer solution level was low in the developer tanks, only the lower part of each of these three films was properly developed. Always check for proper solution depth in developer and fixer tanks before developing your radiographs.

DEVELOPER SOLUTION LEVEL ARTIFACTS   **Plate 84**

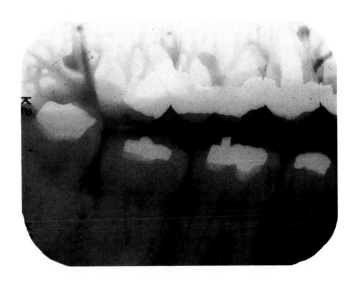

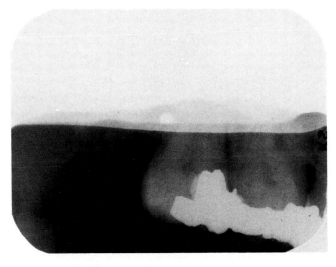

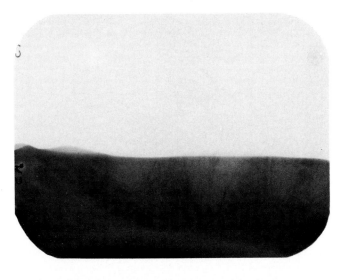

Plate 85   ELONGATED IMAGE; RADIOPAQUE IMAGE; FILM PLACEMENT

   A.   Due to a reduced positive vertical angulation, these teeth appear elongated. This effect is the opposite of foreshortening.
   B.   The operator forgot to remove the patient's maxillary gold partial denture. The large radiopaque area represents the image of the denture.
   C.   When the film was placed in the mouth, it was not positioned far enough down to include the roots of the teeth. If a film holder is used, this is not likely to occur.
   D.   This film was curved when the patient closed down on the film holder. The radiopaque image at the top of this film is that of the metal film holder.

ELONGATED IMAGE; RADIOPAQUE IMAGE; FILM PLACEMENT   **Plate 85**

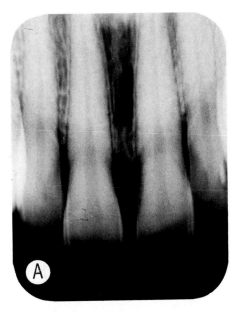

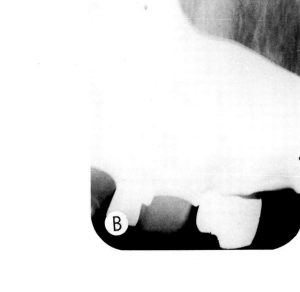

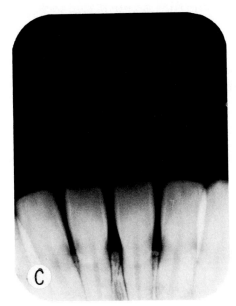

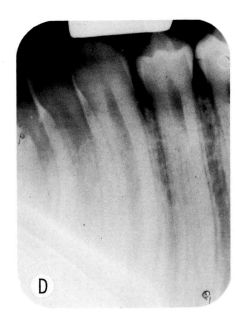

Plate 86   REVERSED FILM; CONE CUT; EYEGLASS ARTIFACT

A.   When placed in the patient's mouth, this film was reversed. The film's tab was facing the lingual aspect of the teeth. The "tire track" design on the film is actually the image of the lead foil that is in the film packet. Radiation has passed through the lead foil, not only leaving its impression on the film but also causing the radiograph to appear too light.

B.   The same thing has happened to this radiograph. The lead foil design looks a little different, but it is still due to the film's being placed backward in the patient's mouth.

C.   The crowns have been obliterated by a cone cut.

D.   The operator failed to remove the patient's eyeglasses, accounting for the large radiopaque area over the apices of the premolars.

REVERSED FILM; CONE CUT; EYEGLASS ARTIFACT   **Plate 86**

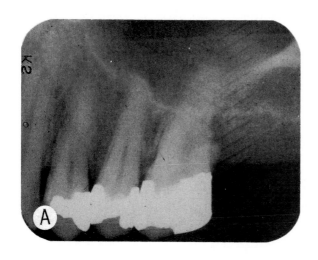

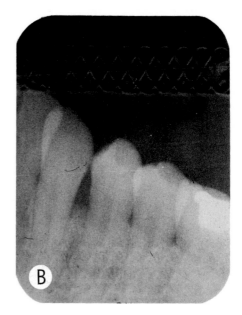

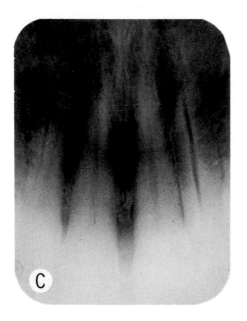

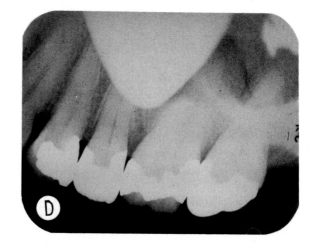

Plate 87   EXPOSURE PROBLEMS; MOTION; DOUBLE IMAGE; FORESHORTENED
IMAGES

A.   Exposing a radiograph to more radiation than is needed (overexposure) will cause the film to appear too dark after development. That is probably the problem with this radiograph. This result could also occur if the film is developed too long or if too high a kilovoltage is used.

B.   The appearance of motion in this radiograph might be due to film motion, patient motion, or excessive x-ray cone motion during the time the film was exposed to radiation.

C.   You are seeing double in this radiograph. The operator accidentally exposed this radiograph twice, thus producing two sets of dental images.

D.   These images are foreshortened. Excessive positive vertical angulation of the x-ray cone produces this effect; insufficient positive vertical angulation causes elongation.

EXPOSURE PROBLEMS; MOTION; DOUBLE IMAGE; FORESHORTENED   **Plate 87**
IMAGES

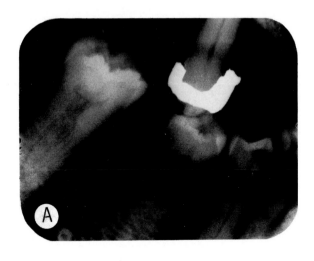

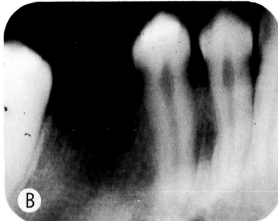

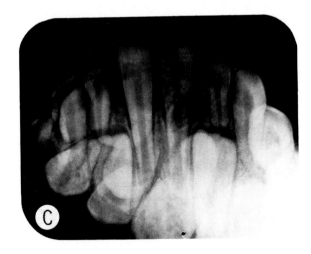

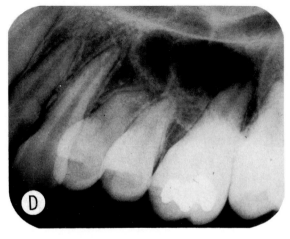

Plate 88   PROCESSING AND POSITIONING ERRORS; CONE CUT; OVERLAPPING

A.   Superimposed over the mesial root of the first molar is a chemical artifact, not a dental lesion. This is due to dried fixer that had remained on the film hanger clip and contaminated the film during development. Film hangers should be thoroughly washed in water before they are used.

B.   When film is improperly positioned in the patient's mouth, a poor radiograph results. The film should have been placed far enough posterior for the third molar to be entirely visible.

C.   This appearance is classified as a posterior cone cut because the cone cut is posterior to the most distal molar.

D.   If horizontal angulation of the x-ray cone had been properly set, overlapping of these interproximals would likely not have occurred.

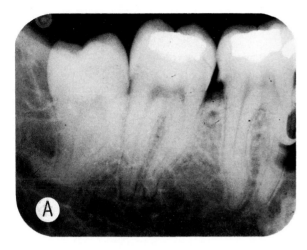

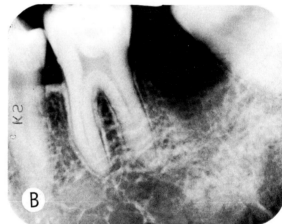

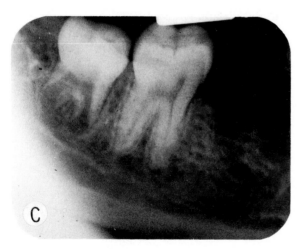

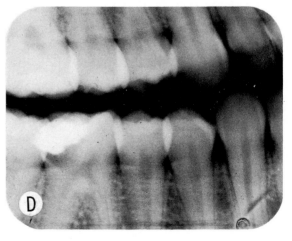

Plate 89   PROCESSING ERRORS; UNAVOIDABLE FILM ARTIFACTS

A.   This film was placed in developer at an elevated temperature. When removed from the developer the film was allowed to dry before it was placed in rinse water. Dried developer spots now mottle the film.

B.   The white streaks on this film are due to fixer solution contamination.

C.   The white vertical lines seen along the edges of this film are due to folding of the film packet. Folding is sometimes necessary if the film is too large for the patient's mouth.

D.   The film emulsion has been scratched. When the film is processed in the manual processor, the soft emulsion is easily scratched in the processing tanks.

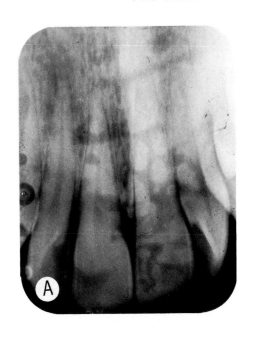

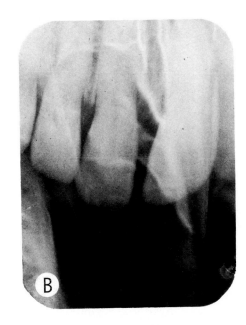

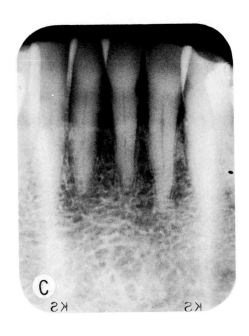

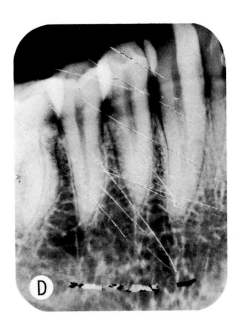

Plate 90   OVERLAPPING; CONE CUTS

A.   Overlapping of tooth contacts interferes with proper interpretation of inter-proximal details.

B.   An anterior film cone cut is a technical error.

C.   Improper horizontal angulation of the x-ray equipment cone can cause image overlapping like that seen in this film.

D.   This is commonly called a superior film cone cut.

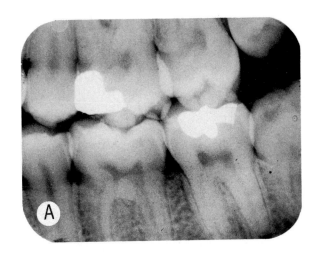

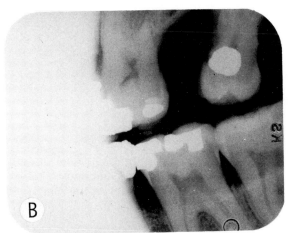

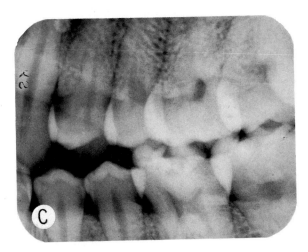

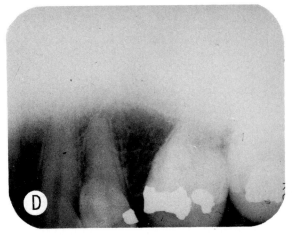

Plate 91   DOUBLE AND REVERSED IMAGE; DEVELOPER ARTIFACT

A.   Occlusal films are sometimes double-exposed. The film packet was also placed backward in the patient's mouth. Notice the "tire tracks" from the lead foil backing in the film packet.

B.   The black spots on the film are developer solution stains. There also appear to be two supernumerary teeth developing in the palate.

DOUBLE AND REVERSED IMAGE; DEVELOPER ARTIFACT Plate 91

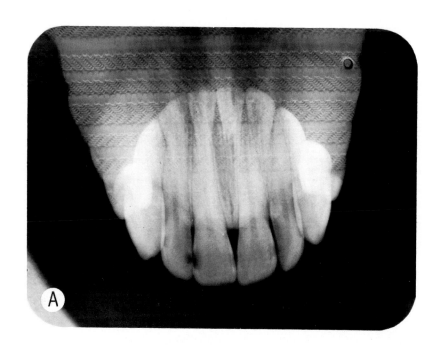

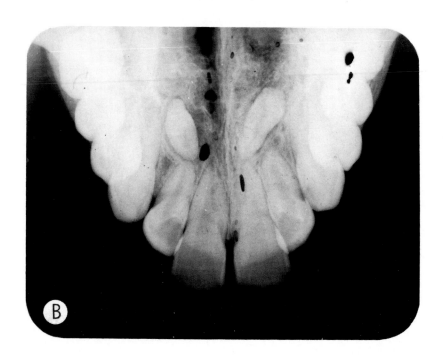

Plate 92   OPAQUE ARTIFACTS (PROCESSING ERROR)

The operator did not remove the inner paper wrapping surrounding the film. When the film was processed, air was trapped between the film and the paper surfaces. Those areas that were not properly developed appear as opaque artifacts.

OPAQUE ARTIFACTS (PROCESSING ERROR) **Plate 92**

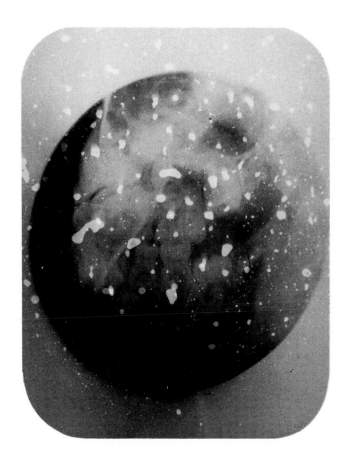

Plate 93   PROCESSING ERRORS

A.   A fingerprint can be seen over the roots of the premolars. The operator's hands had been exposed to fluoride solution and were not washed before developing this film. Developer solution could cause this same artifact.

B.   This is one of two films that adhered to each other during the developing and fixing process. The film cannot be improved because the emulsion has been damaged.

C.   During processing of this film, another film overlapped it. This is the reason you see a line through the molars. Fixer was accidentally spilled on this film before it was developed. This is evidenced by the opaque spots on the mesial root apices of the first and second molars.

D.   When developer solution is smeared on a film prior to development, this is the usual result.

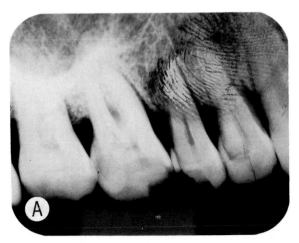

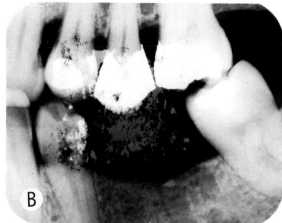

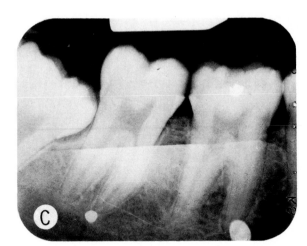

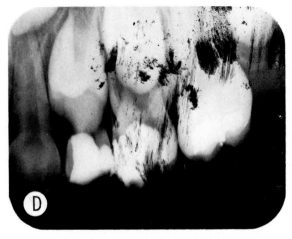

Plate 94   CHEMICAL SPILLS; PACKAGING ARTIFACT

A.   There are black dots on this film. They were caused by developer solution that was accidentally spilled on the film before developing.

B.   The white images that appear on the roots of these teeth are drops of fixer solution, which was accidentally spilled on the film before it was developed.

C.   The large black area on this film was caused by developer solution being splashed on the film before developing.

D.   This is an unusual packaging artifact that is very likely caused by the inner black paper covering the film.

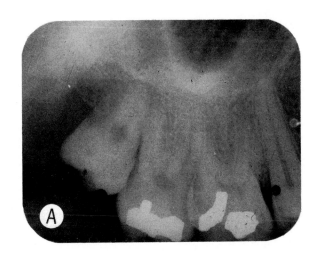

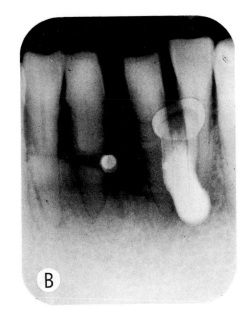

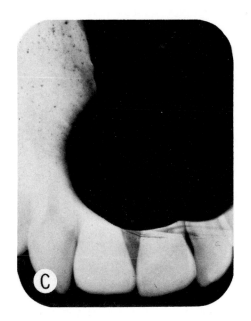

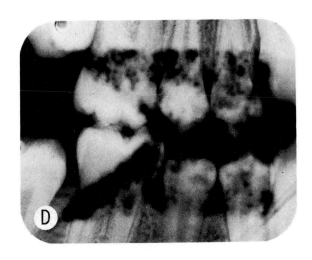

SECTION FOUR

ITEMS COMMONLY SEEN IN DENTAL RADIOGRAPHS

Plate 95   RUBBERBAND IMAGES

If you look closely at these three radiographs, you will see the slightly radiopaque images of rubberbands (white arrowheads). They were wrapped around cotton rolls and film holders when these radiographs were taken.

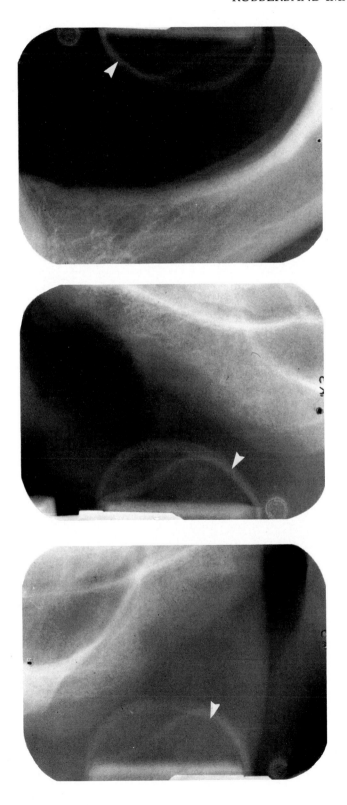

Plate 96   SALIVARY GLAND DEPRESSION

The large round radiolucency seen in these three mandibular radiographs is known as the salivary gland depression phenomenon.

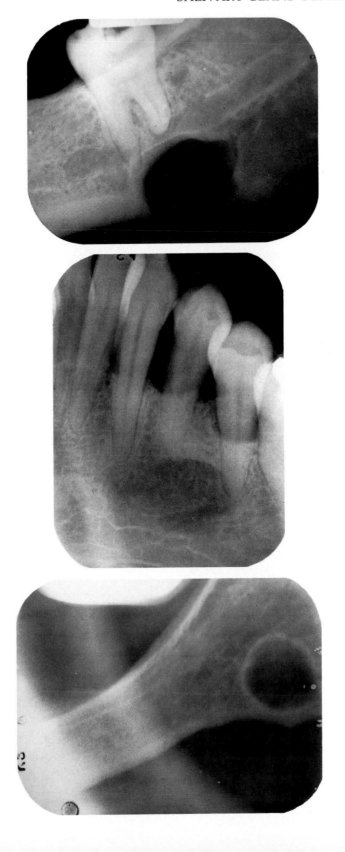

Plate 97   ROOT FRACTURE; MALFORMED UNERUPTED TOOTH; RETAINED TOOTH REMNANT; INVERTED THIRD MOLAR; MUCOUS RETENTION CYST (MUCOCELE)

These five intraoral radiographs each show interesting entities.

A.   The root of the maxillary left central incisor is fractured.
B.   An unerupted lateral incisor that appears to be malformed.
C.   A retained primary tooth remnant (black arrowhead). The tooth remnant is still attached to the gingival soft tissue.
D.   An inverted third molar, which is located distal to the second molar.
E.   A dome-shaped mucous retention cyst (mucocele) superimposed over the roots of the first molar.

ROOT FRACTURE; MALFORMED UNERUPTED TOOTH; RETAINED TOOTH **Plate 97**
REMNANT; INVERTED THIRD MOLAR; MUCOUS RETENTION CYST
(MUCOCELE)

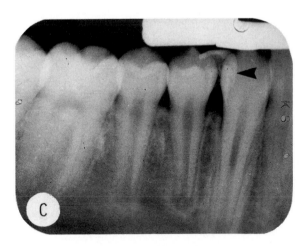

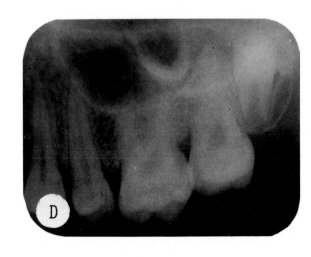

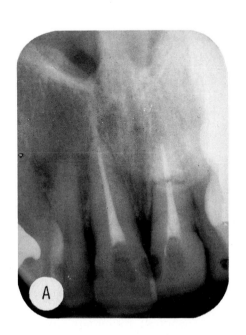

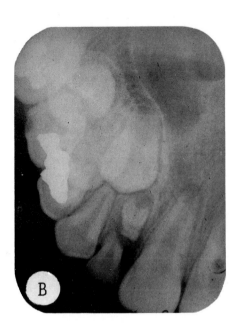

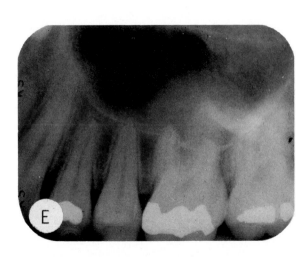

Plate 98   MICRODONT; PERIAPICAL RADIOLUCENCY; CARIES; ENDODONTICS; RETROGRADE SILVER ALLOYS; ROOT RESORPTION; MALFORMED CROWN

A.   The microdont lateral incisor seen in this film is cariously involved; also, a periapical radiolucency indicating pathology is located there. The central incisor has a large distal carious lesion, whereas the canine appears to have a large coronal carious lesion.

B.   These teeth had been endodontically treated and also have retrograde silver alloys. Both teeth have undergone root resorption. The patient is 25 years of age.

C.   The lateral incisor in this film may have been injured during its early developmental stage. That may be the reason for the malformed crown.

MICRODONT; PERIAPICAL RADIOLUCENCY; CARIES; ENDODONTICS; RETROGRADE SILVER ALLOYS; ROOT RESORPTION; MALFORMED CROWN

Plate 98

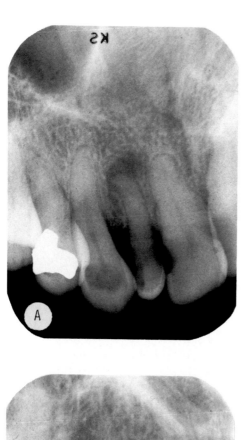

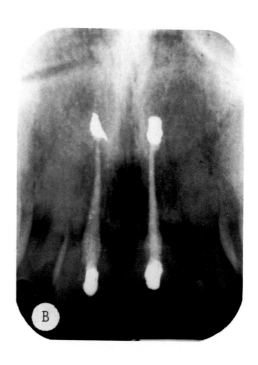

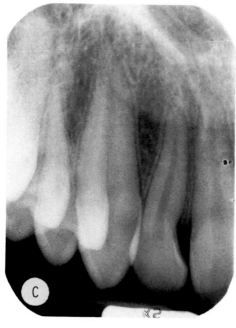

Plate 99   METAL PARTIAL DENTURE; IODOFORM GAUZE

A. This film shows the result of leaving a metal partial denture in the patient's mouth when taking an intraoral radiograph. Removable appliances should be removed prior to taking intraoral radiographs.

B. If you look carefully you can see, distal to the second molar, the lightly opaque image of iodoform gauze. This was inadvertently left in the third molar extraction site.

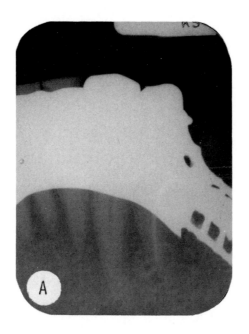

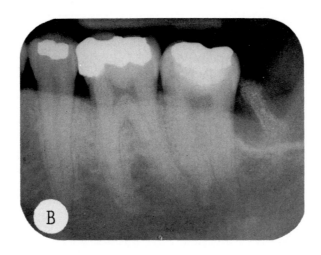

Plate 100   CANTILEVERED BRIDGE PONTIC; INTERNAL RESORPTION, CROWN FRACTURE; PERIAPICAL RADIOLUCENCY; ROOT RESORPTION

A.   The first permanent premolar has been replaced with a cantilevered bridge pontic.

B.   This film was taken in a male patient who at 13 years of age sustained a traumatic blow to his maxillary anterior teeth. Now, at the age of 16 years there is internal resorption, fracture of the crown, and a periapical radiolucency of the left central incisor. Also, note the root resorption.

CANTILEVERED BRIDGE PONTIC; INTERNAL RESORPTION, CROWN **Plate 100**
FRACTURE; PERIAPICAL RADIOLUCENCY; ROOT RESORPTION

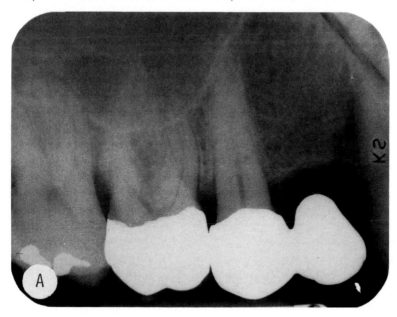

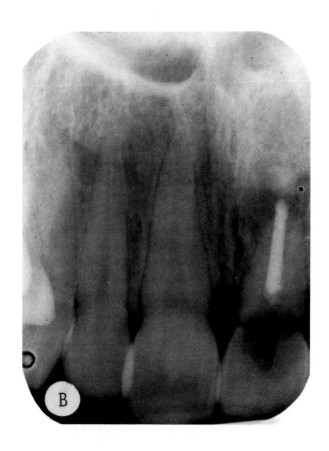

Plate 101   LEAD PELLET; BULLET IN SINUS

A.   This patient is 19 years old. When he was 6 years old, he was accidentally shot in the mouth with a lead pellet. The lead pellet is located in the soft tissue of the cheek superimposed over the first premolar.

B.   This panoramic view is that of a male patient who was accidentally shot. The bullet lodged in the maxillary left sinus (black arrowhead). Note the scattered radiopaque metal fragments around the right and left palatal areas.

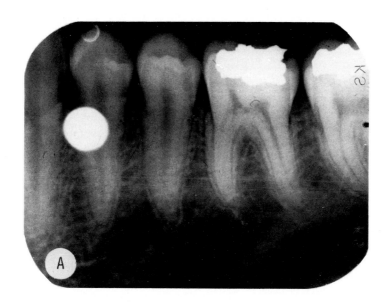

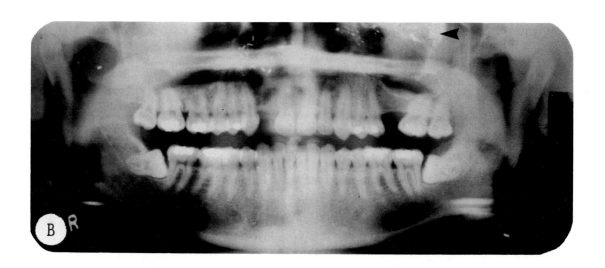

Plate 102   INCISIVE NERVE FORAMEN CYST (NASOPALATINE FORAMEN CYST);
TONGUE

A.   The large radiolucency in the maxilla of this film is an incisive nerve foramen cyst. It is also called a nasopalatine foramen cyst.

B.   The black arrowhead is pointing at the image of the patient's tongue. Part of the tongue became superimposed over the film when this radiograph was taken.

INCISIVE NERVE FORAMEN CYST (NASOPALATINE FORAMEN CYST); TONGUE

Plate 102

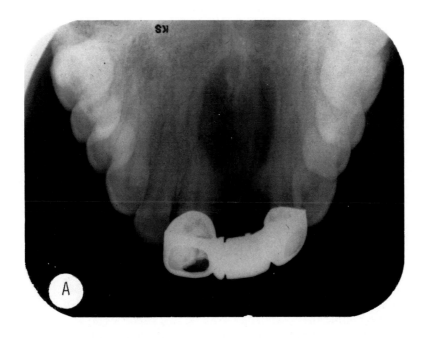

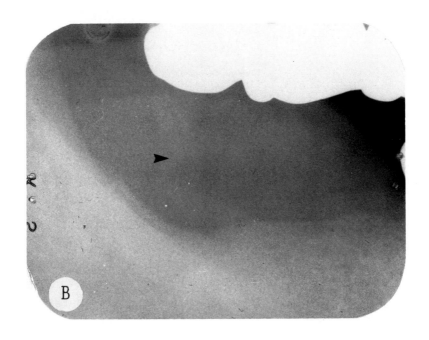

Plate 103   FALSE FRACTURE ARTIFACT; NASAL BONE FRACTURE

A.   The right mandibular body appears to be fractured (white arrowhead). Actually, the patient moved during the exposure of the right side, thus producing this false artifact, which does resemble a fracture of the jaw.

B.   Close observation will reveal a fracture of the nasal bone (white arrowhead). The patient was accidentally hit in the nose during a baseball game.

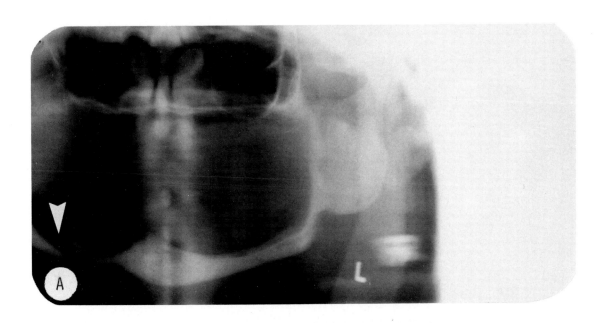

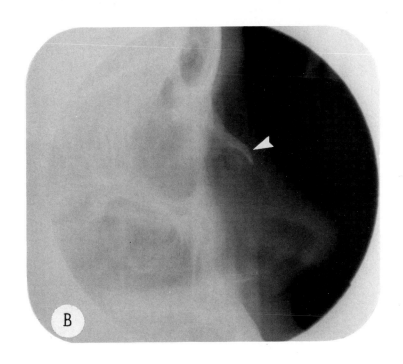

Plate 104   CALCIFIED STYLOHYOID LIGAMENTS

Look at all three of these panoramic films. The black arrowheads are pointing at calcified stylohyoid ligaments.

CALCIFIED STYLOHYOID LIGAMENTS   **Plate 104**

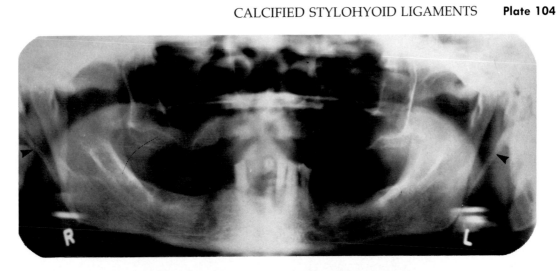

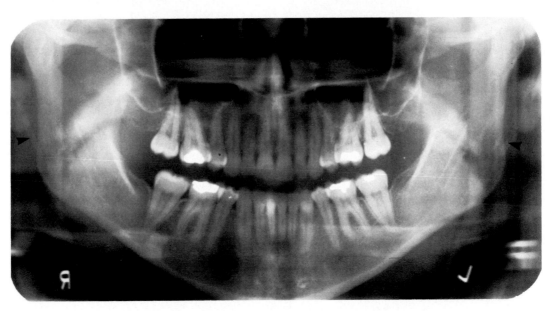

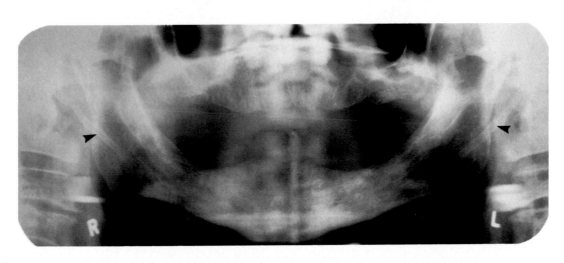

Plate 105   DENTIGEROUS CYST

The large radiolucency in the left mandible surrounding the molar tooth is a dentigerous cyst.

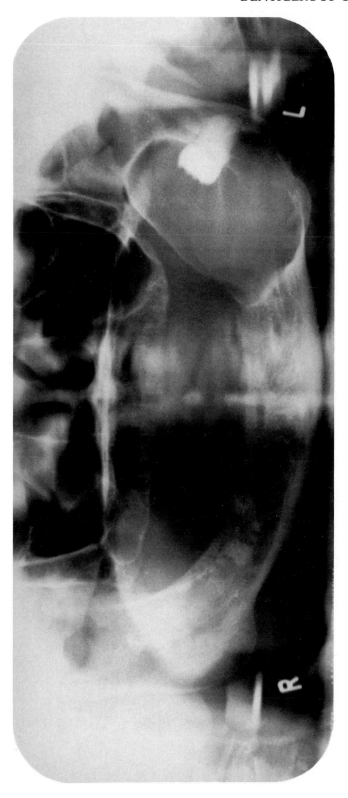

Plate 106   SUPERNUMERARY MOLARS

A and B.   There are supernumerary molars in both of these panoramic views. In **A** there are five maxillary molars in the right quadrant. There are four in the left quadrant. In **B** there are four molars in each of the four quadrants.

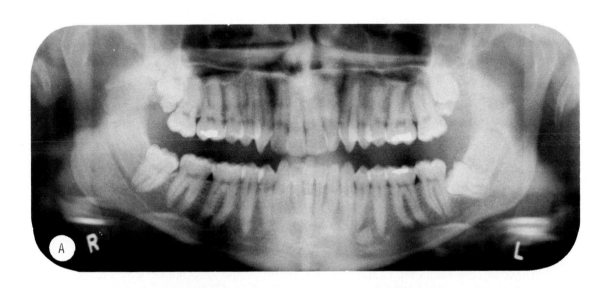

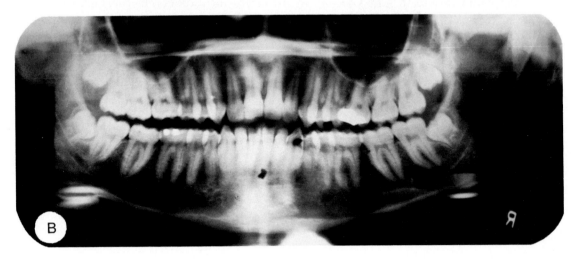

Plate 107   SUPERNUMERARY TEETH

These are the radiographs and intraoral photographs of a patient with eleven supernumerary teeth. Can you find them? Check the radiographs carefully.

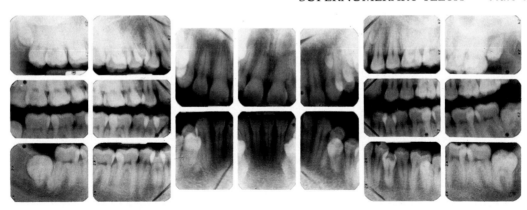

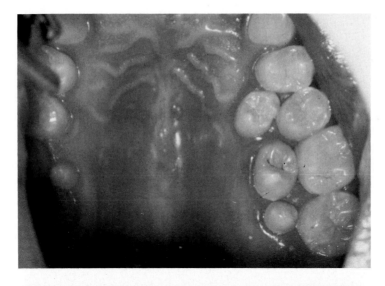

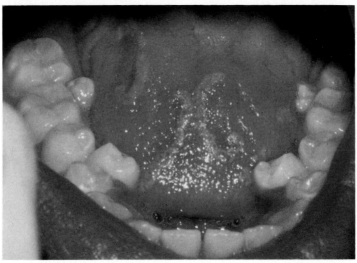

Plate 108   PORCELAIN; METAL ARTIFACTS

A. The porcelain sanitary pontic shows up well on this radiograph. The radiopaque spot under the pontic is most likely silver alloy.

B. If you look closely at the radiopaque object you can recognize the tip of a dental bur.

C. All of the radiopaque spots represent metal fragments from a shotgun injury. The fragments are in the patient's cheek.

D. The radiopaque object superimposed over the second molar is a metal clasp that is attached to an acrylic partial denture (the acrylic partial denture does not show radiographically).

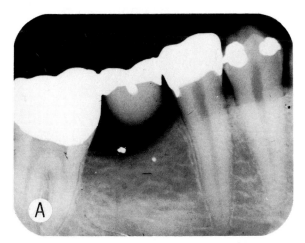

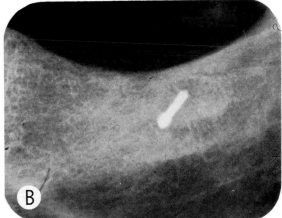

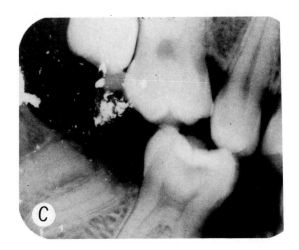

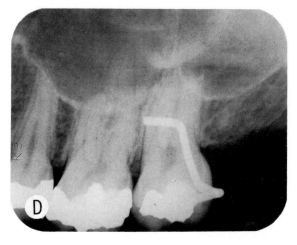

Plate 109 IMPLANT; CANTILEVERED BRIDGE; DILACERATED ROOTS; RESORBED ROOTS

A. This is a blade implant used as an abutment for a bridge.
B. This four-unit bridge has a distal cantilevered unit.
C. The second and third molars have roots that have undergone severe dilaceration.
D. The distal root of the first molar has resorbed, and it appears that the pulp chamber and canals have calcified.

IMPLANT; CANTILEVERED BRIDGE; DILACERATED ROOTS; RESORBED ROOTS

Plate 109

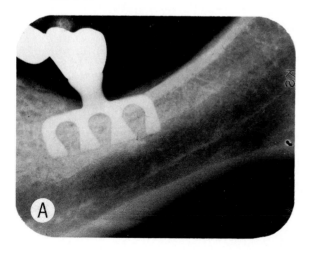

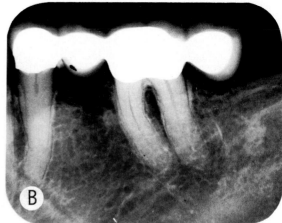

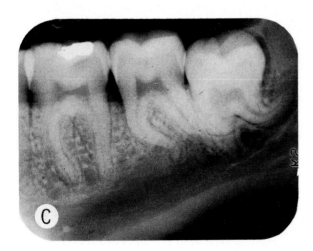

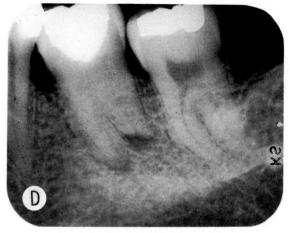

Plate 110   PINS; POST AND CORE; RETROGRADE ALLOYS

A.   A stainless steel pin was placed in the second molar. It is a mystery why the pin was placed.

B.   The gold post and core restoration was too broad. It also does not follow the canal, which was endodontically treated. Oxyphosphate cement used to fix the post and core restoration is seen leaking laterally through the fractured portion of the tooth.

C.   The retrograde silver alloy missed its mark at the apex of the right central incisor.

D.   The endodontic treatment in the first premolar looks good, but something went wrong with the attempted retrograde silver alloy restoration.

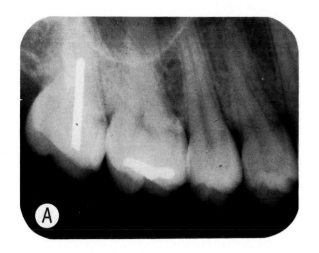

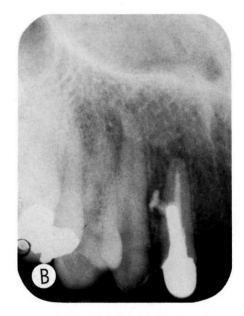

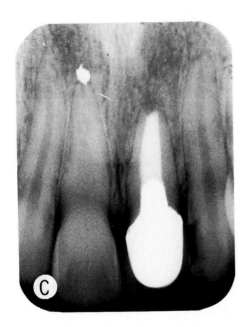

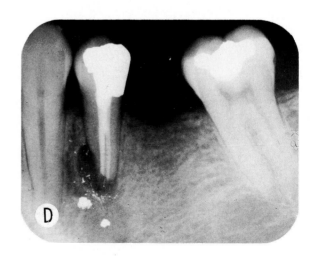

A.   The facial and lingual surfaces of the appliance cemented in the root canals of these teeth were covered with a resin material. The dark radiolucent areas surrounding the apices of the teeth indicate loss of bone, a pathologic development resulting from infection of the teeth.

B.   The canine demonstrates no pulp chamber. Diffuse calcification is a good description of this condition.

C.   The lingual access opening into the pulp chamber of the left central incisor is particularly evident from the large radiolucency in the crown.

D.   An endodontic stabilizer pin was used to anchor this tooth root in the bone.

UNUSUAL FINDINGS; CALCIFIED PULP CHAMBER; RADIOLUCENCIES; **Plate 111**
STABILIZER PIN

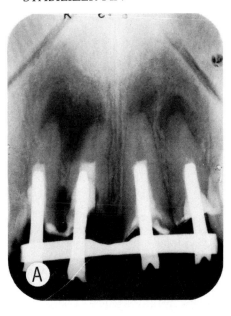

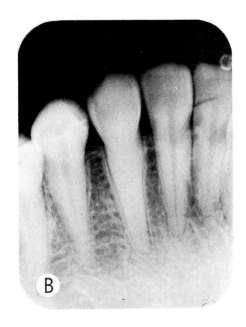

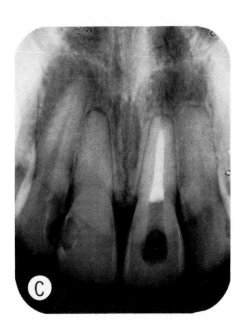

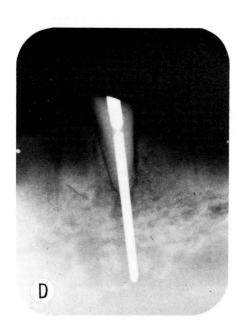

Plate 112   RESTORATIONS; RECURRENT CARIES; IMPEDED PREMOLAR ERUPTION

A.   A silver alloy restoration was placed in the first molar. Recurrent caries is
          evident. The radiopaque line just superior to the pulp chamber is secondary
          dentin.

B.   Reinforcing pins were placed in the right lateral incisor and both central
          incisors. They were used to reinforce their respective resin restorations. There
          is a large pathosis apical to the left lateral incisor, which has been endodontically
          treated and then fitted with a gold post and core.

C.   The lateral incisor has a poorly crafted retrograde silver alloy restoration.

D.   The second premolar is not likely to erupt normally. There is a copper band
          located just occlusal to the second premolar. You can barely see the remnants
          of the second primary molar inside the copper band.

RESTORATIONS; RECURRENT CARIES; IMPEDED PREMOLAR ERUPTION Plate 112

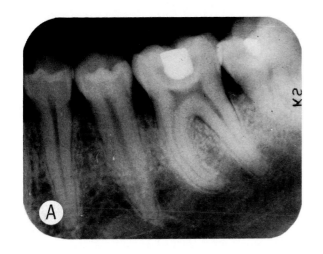

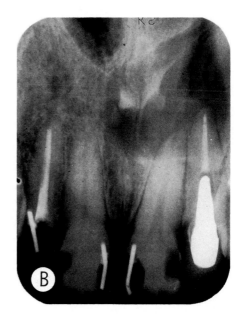

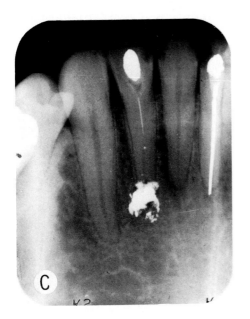

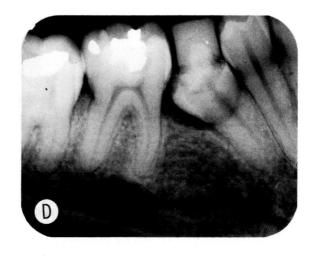

Plate 113   MUCOCELE; SUPERNUMERARY TOOTH; MICRODONT; EXTRUDED TEETH

A.   The semicircular gray area in the maxillary sinus is a mucocele. The more radiopaque object at the top of the film is the zygomatic process.

B.   Between the roots of the maxillary second premolar and molar is a developing supernumerary tooth.

C.   Just distal to the molar is a microdont.

D.   These teeth are extruded (overerupted). They have no opposing teeth in the mandible. Note the calculus between the molars.

MUCOCELE; SUPERNUMERARY TOOTH; MICRODONT; EXTRUDED TEETH   **Plate 113**

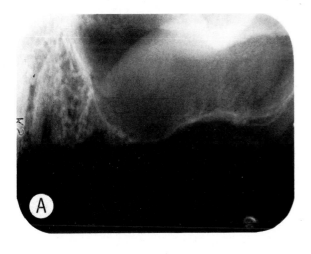

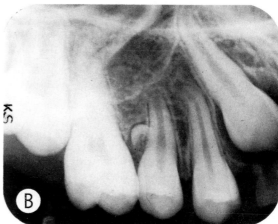

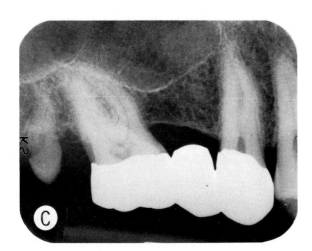

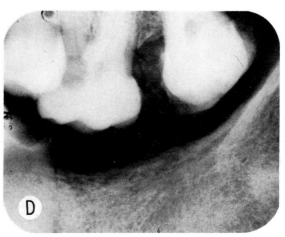

Plate 114   METALLIC ARTIFACTS

A.   It appears that some silver alloy has become wedged between the crown of the horizontal molar and the distal root of the erect molar.

B.   A reinforcing pin has accidentally penetrated through the mesial-cervical aspect of the maxillary second premolar.

C.   The radiopaque material just distal to the distal root of the second molar is a wire used to reduce a bone fracture.

D.   That radiopaque object in the bone is a piece of metal. No one seems to know how it got there.

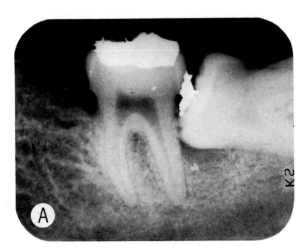

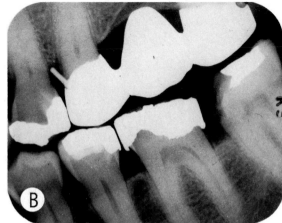

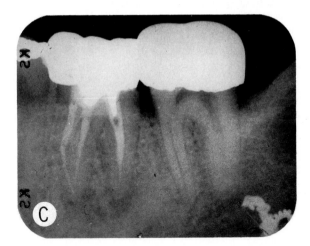

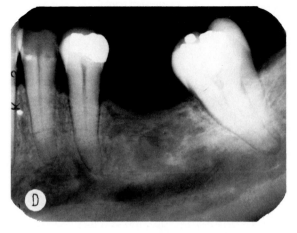

Plate 115   DENS IN DENTE (DENS INVAGINATUS); CALCIFIED PULP CHAMBER AND CANAL; LINGUAL FORAMEN AND CANAL; CEMENTOMA (PERIAPICAL CEMENTAL DYSPLASIA)

A.   The lateral incisor has a developmental defect called dens invaginatus (dens in dente).

B.   Radiographically neither the pulp chamber nor the canal is revealed in the canine. Calcific metamorphosis has closed the pulp chamber and canal.

C.   There are no permanent lateral incisors. Note the lingual foramen and the lingual canal.

D.   These teeth were vital. The apical radiolucency with a calcified area in the center is periapical cemental dysplasia (cementoma).

DENS IN DENTE (DENS INVAGINATUS); CALCIFIED PULP CHAMBER AND CANAL; LINGUAL FORAMEN AND CANAL; CEMENTOMA (PERIAPICAL CEMENTAL DYSPLASIA)

Plate 115

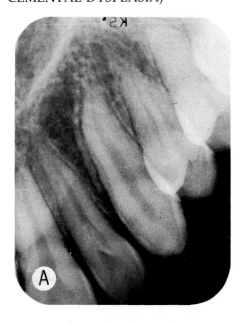

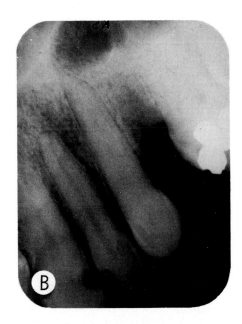

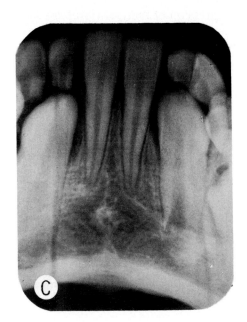

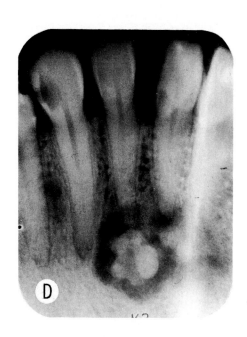

Plate 116   EXTRACTION SITE; CHANGES IN LAMINA DURA; RUBBER-BASE
MATERIAL

A.   The extraction site of the second premolar is evident. The radiopaque lamina
dura is distinct.

B.   The same extraction site has almost completely calcified several months later.
The lamina dura is no longer distinct.

C.   The second premolar has been prepared for a full-crown restoration. A rubber-
base elastic material was used to make an impression of the tooth preparation.

D.   Just distal to the prepared tooth is a radiopaque object that actually was a piece
of the rubber-base material used to make an impression of the tooth preparation.
The material appeared to leak into the gingival sulcus. It was removed without
any postoperative problem.

EXTRACTION SITE; CHANGES IN LAMINA DURA; RUBBER-BASE MATERIAL Plate 116

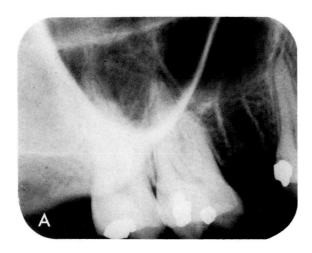

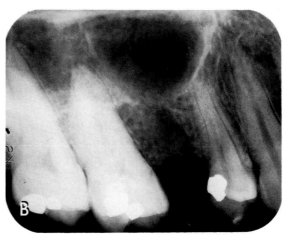

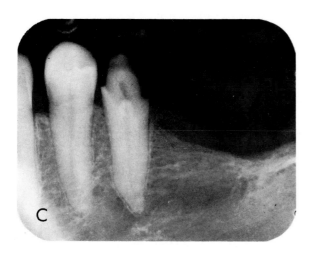

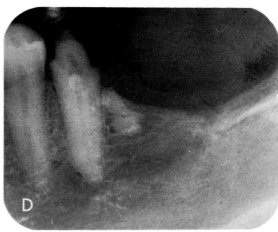

Plate 117   TAURODONT; CHRONIC DIFFUSE SCLEROSING OSTEOMYELITIS

A.   Both of these radiographs are from the same patient. The teeth demonstrate the typical form of taurodonts (or taurodontism).

B.   Both radiographs are from the same patient and demonstrate chronic diffuse sclerosing osteomyelitis.

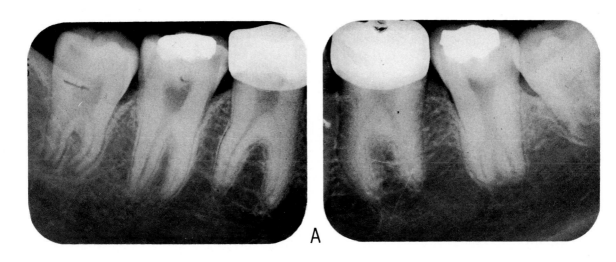

A

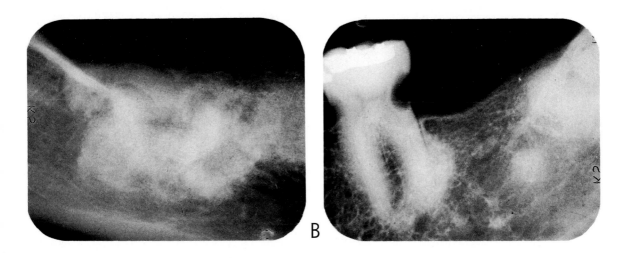

B

Plate 118   ACRYLIC BRIDGE; ACRYLIC DENTURE

   A.   These two radiographs are from the same individual. The canines have been prepared for full-crown restorations, and a temporary acrylic bridge has been placed to maintain the space.
   B.   A maxillary acrylic denture was left in the mouth when these bitewing radiographs were made.

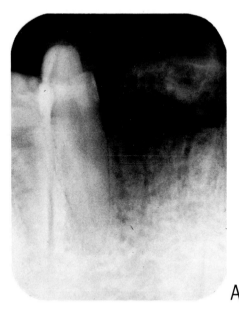
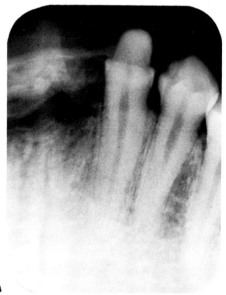

A

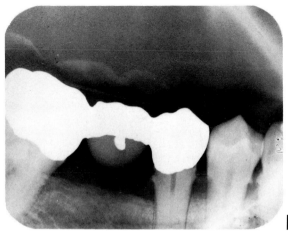
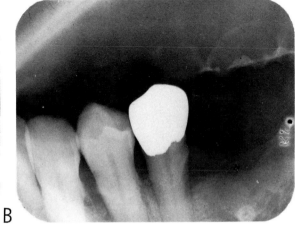

B

Plate 119 RADIOPAQUE MATERIALS; BIFID ROOTS

A.   The radiopaque objects lodged in the alveolus of the extracted second premolar are trapped silver alloy chips from restorations that were already in the first premolar. When the first premolar was prepared for its ceramic-fused-to-gold restoration, the silver alloy chips fell into the then unhealed alveolus.

B.   The patient was in an automobile accident. The large opaque object located apical to the teeth is a piece of leaded automobile glass.

C.   This premolar has an unusual bifid root formation.

D.   The canine also has an unusual bifid root formation.

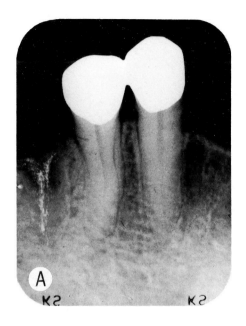

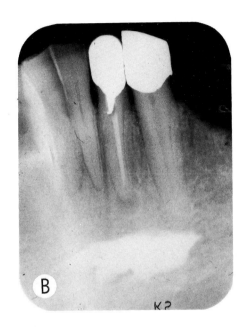

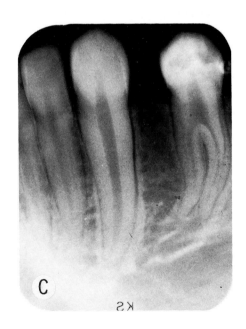

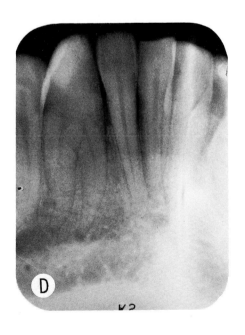

Plate 120   RESORPTION; OVERHANG; WOODEN HOLDERS; COTTON ROLLS

A.   The mesial root of the first molar has undergone much resorption. Note the mesial overhang of the restoration, which is causing the alveolar bone loss.

B.   The square, slightly opaque image at the top of the film is part of a wooden film holder. The visible image between the film holder and the alveolar ridge is a cotton roll.

C.   The third molar has apparently been impacted in bone for some time. It appears to be undergoing resorption. Note the mottled appearance of the crown.

D.   Between the wooden film holder and the alveolar ridge is the slightly opaque image of a cotton roll.

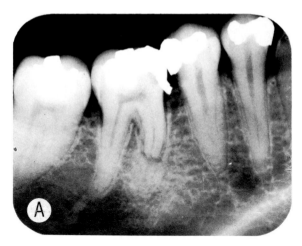

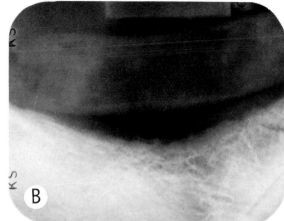

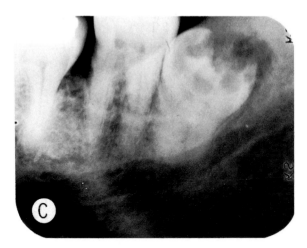

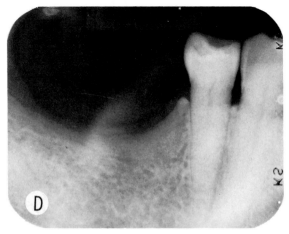

Plate 121 IMPACTION; CROSS-FIRE VIEW; LATERAL FACIAL VIEW

A. An occlusal radiograph revealed the right central incisor impaction located near the nasal fossa.

B. A cross-fire occlusal film was made in an attempt to locate the labial or palatal position of the tooth. As you see, this film does not show the tooth's location.

C. This lateral facial film clearly shows the location of the tooth beneath the nasal fossa.

IMPACTION; CROSS-FIRE VIEW; LATERAL FACIAL VIEW   **Plate 121**

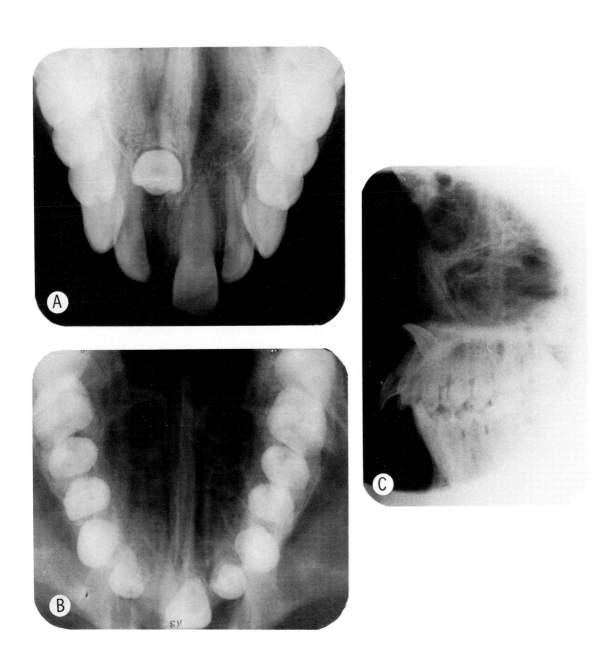

Plate 122   IMPACTION; CALCULUS; LANDMARKS; WORN GOLD CROWN

A. The second primary molar remained in the maxillary arch. The second permanent premolar was not able to erupt properly and became impacted.

B. This molar is covered with calculus.

C. The maxillary tuberosity and the maxillary sinus are quite visible. An unusually long coronoid process is also visible.

D. The dark spot seen on the crown of the first premolar is a worn surface of the gold crown.

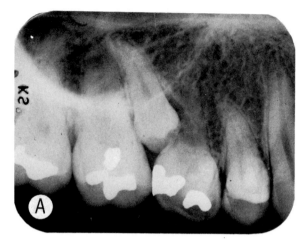

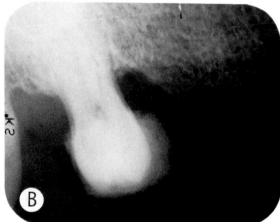

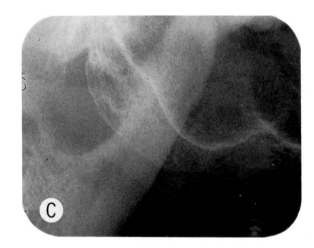

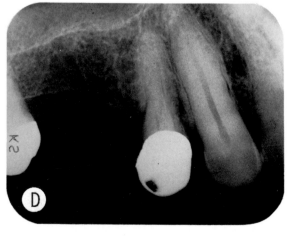

Plate 123   MANDIBULAR TORI

The large areas of radiopacity seen superimposed over the roots of these teeth are lingual mandibular tori.

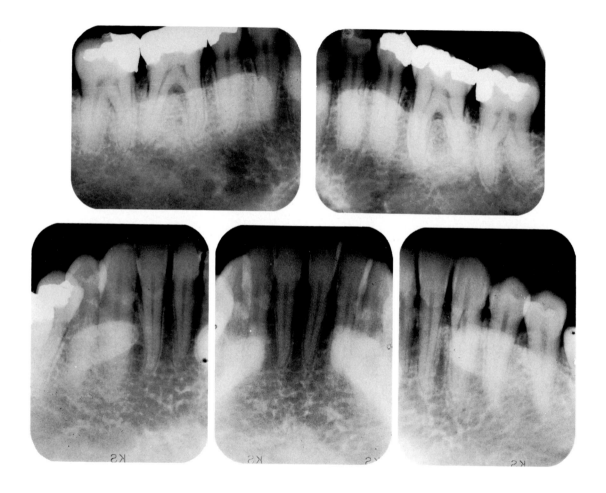

Plate 124   MAXILLARY TORUS

Both of these radiographs were taken in the same patient. The black arrowheads indicate the location of a large maxillary torus.

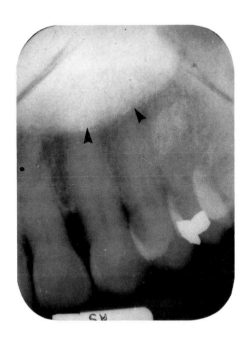

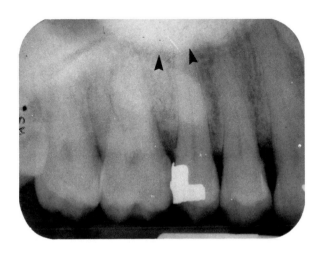

Plate 125   MAXILLARY/MANDIBULAR TORI

This panoramic radiograph and the accompanying intraoral radiographic series will help you locate the various maxillary and mandibular tori in this patient's oral cavity. The next page shows three clinical intraoral photographic views of this patient's tori. You should be able to locate the areas.

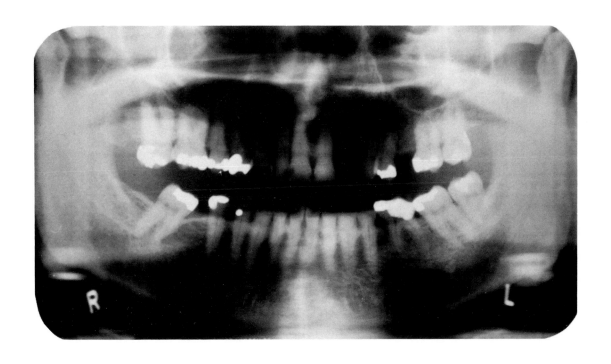

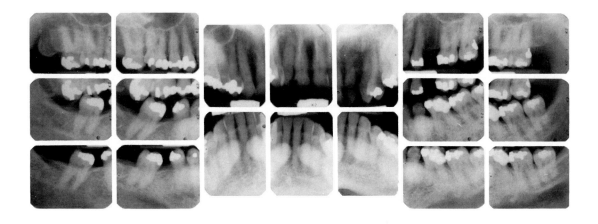

MAXILLARY/MANDIBULAR TORI   **Plate 125**

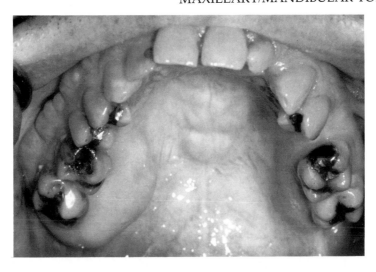

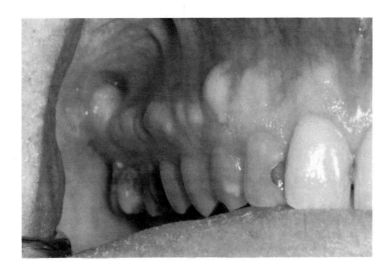

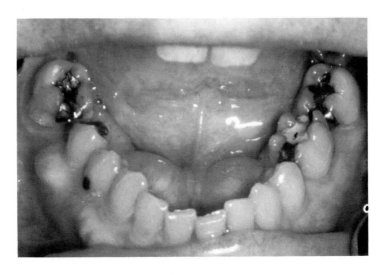

Plate 126   RESTORATIONS; WORN RESTORATIONS

A.   This was a functional three-unit gold bridge until the premolar abutment crown became so worn around the crown that the cervical portion of the crown collapsed in the position in which you now see it.

B.   In order to close the space between these two central incisors, the gold crown restoration was greatly overcontoured.

C.   This restoration was prepared in order to close the existing space between the two teeth. The metal covering the central incisor wore through.

D.   The pontic and distal abutment are all that remain of a three-unit bridge. The anterior bridge unit was lost some time before this radiograph was made.

261

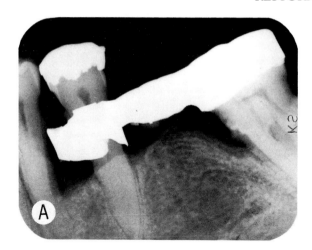

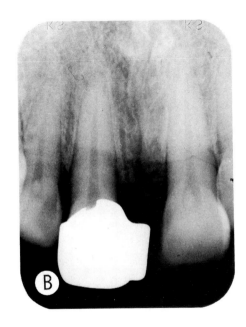

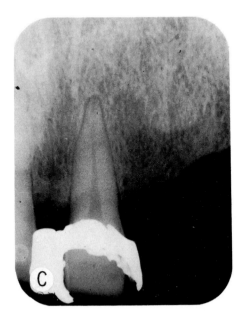

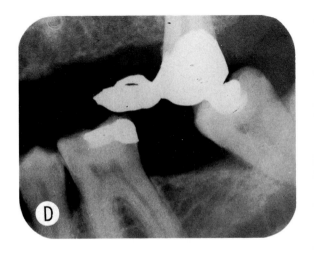

Plate 127   ROOT FRACTURE; MESIODENS; RESORPTION; BONE LOSS

A.   The right maxillary central incisor has a root fracture. Note that the apical third of the root canal appears calcified.

B.   The image seen between the maxillary central incisor roots is of a supernumerary tooth commonly called a mesiodens. The mesiodens appears to be resorbing, as indicated by the radiolucency.

C.   These teeth were endodontically treated. The general radiolucency of these teeth appears to indicate that they are undergoing resorption.

D.   Two poorly contoured crowns have been placed on these central incisors. There is a great deal of alveolar bone loss. Note also the calculus deposits on these teeth.

ROOT FRACTURE; MESIODENS; RESORPTION; BONE LOSS   **Plate 127**

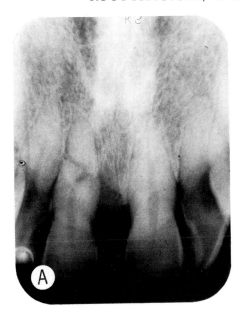

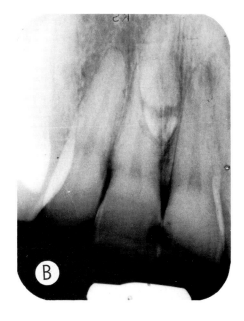

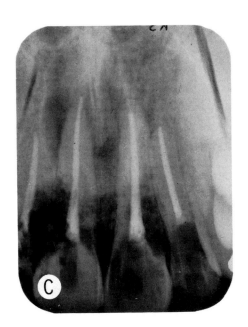

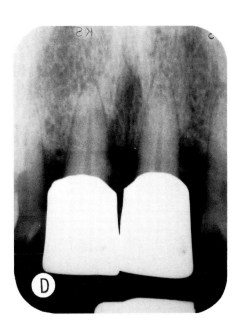

Plate 128   MAXILLARY SINUS RECESS; CARIES; ROOT REMNANTS

A.   The deep radiolucent spot in the maxillary sinus is called the maxillary sinus recess.

B.   The maxillary sinus recess is also seen in this film.

C.   Caries has taken its toll of these teeth. Multiple root remnants are seen in this film.

D.   Several root remnants are seen in the maxillary tuberosity. The coronoid process is just visible on the left of this film.

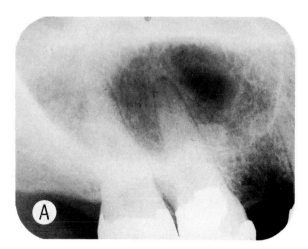

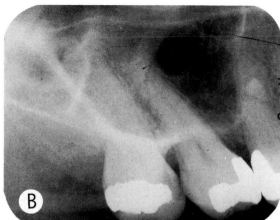

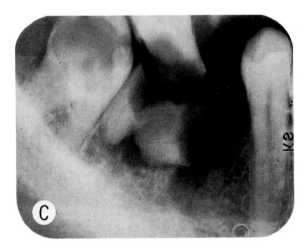

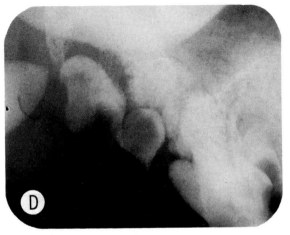

Plate 129   METALLIC ARTIFACT

A. This radiograph was made when the patient appeared at the dental clinic. The radiopaque mass superimposed over the root of the incisor does not appear to be a chemical artifact.

B. As it turns out, another film was placed under the patient's upper lip and this is the result. The radiopaque mass is still there, and it appears to be at the base of the anterior nasal spine. The patient stated that he had sustained an injury in an automobile accident several years earlier. This is either a piece of metal or leaded glass. Note the patient's lip.

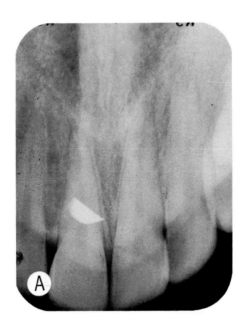

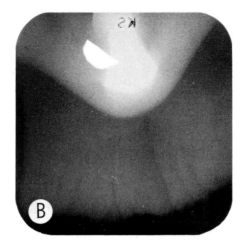

Plate 130　RESTORATIVE MATERIALS

- **A.**　Reinforcing wires have been used in the restoring of the second premolar.
- **B.**　Reinforcing wires have been used to restore the fractured mesial incisal edge of the central incisor.
- **C.**　A vitreous carbon implant was used to replace the lost canine. Vitreous carbon material is radiolucent, but the gold post and core are radiopaque.
- **D.**　These two central incisors were treated with gutta percha. The right incisor has a length of metal tubing that has been placed in the crown. The radiolucent areas seen in the tubing are small holes that have been placed in the tubing to assist with retention of resin restorative material.

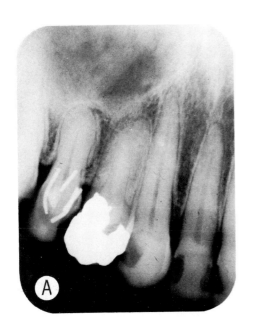

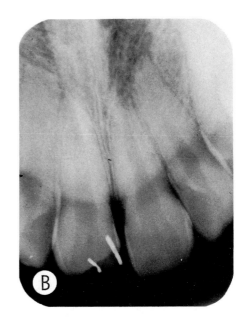

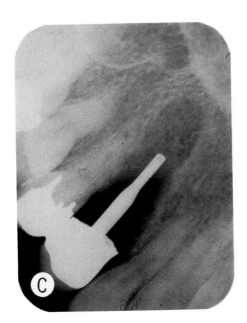

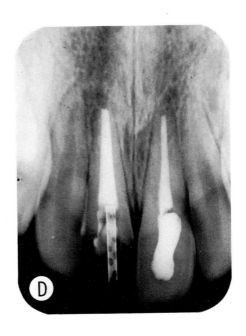

Plate 131   ROOT CARIES

A.   The canine does not appear to be as cariously involved as the other teeth. Cervical caries appears to circle the other teeth and is progressing along the root surfaces.

B.   Cervical caries is progressing along the tooth roots. The two vertical radiopaque lines were caused by bending or creasing of the radiographic film (the film emulsion apparently was not cracked).

C.   The large carious lesions have practically dissected what appears to be a canine tooth.

D.   The mesial root of the second molar and the distal root of the first molar show large carious lesions.

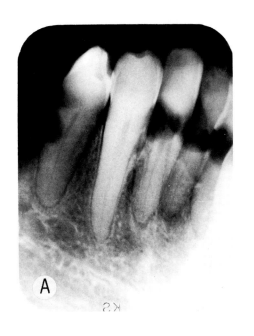

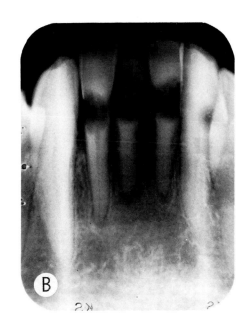

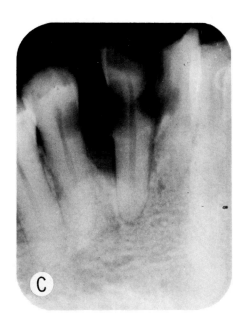

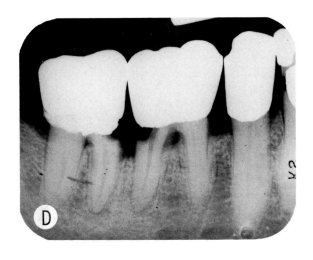

Plate 132   IMPACTION; CALCULUS; CYSTIC LESION

A.   The second premolar is impacted and appears to be undergoing resorption.
B.   Calculus shows up very well at the cervical aspect of these teeth.
C.   Equally clear evidence of calculus is seen in this radiograph.
D.   The second premolar will not be able to erupt normally. There is a lack of
      space between the first premolar and the first molar. The radiolucent area
      around the crown of the unerupted premolar might be a cyst; the tissue in this
      area should be checked by biopsy. The mesial aspect of the unerupted third
      molar can be seen.

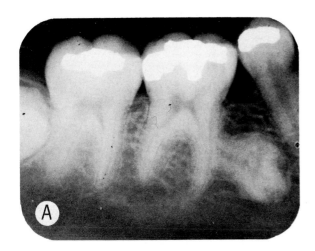

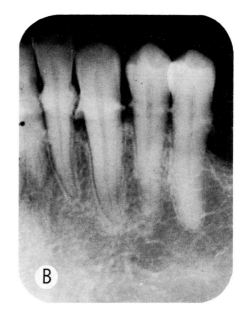

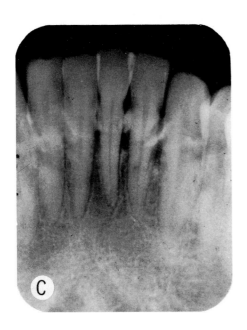

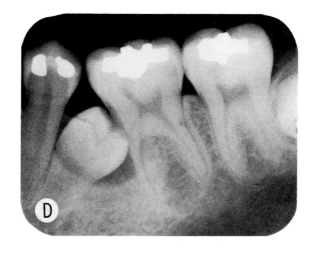

SECTION FIVE

OTHER IMAGING MODALITIES

Plate 133   RADIONUCLIDE SALIVARY GLAND STUDY OF A NORMAL PAROTID
GLAND; RADIONUCLIDE STUDY OF A WARTHIN'S TUMOR IN A
PAROTID GLAND

A.   The images in this film are those of a radionuclide salivary gland study. This
study demonstrates normal uptake by the parotid salivary gland (black arrowheads) at 5 and 10 minutes following radionuclide injection.

B.   This radionuclide salivary gland study shows increased uptake in the lower
pole of the left parotid gland (black arrowheads). This was due to a Warthin's
tumor. (A and B courtesy of Dr. Angelo DelBalso.)

RADIONUCLIDE SALIVARY GLAND STUDY OF A NORMAL PAROTID
GLAND; RADIONUCLIDE STUDY OF A WARTHIN'S TUMOR IN A
PAROTID GLAND

Plate 133

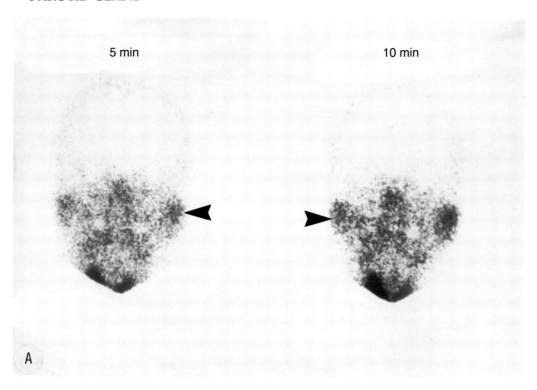

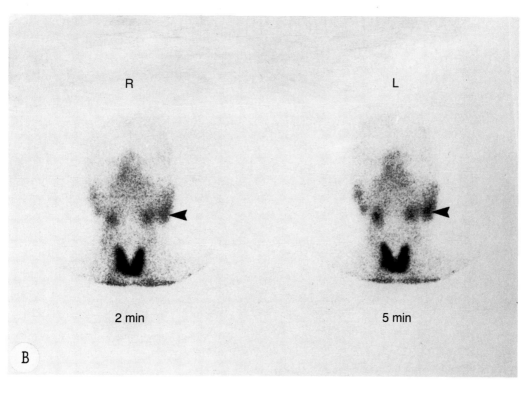

Plate 134   SONOGRAM OF A MIXED TUMOR; RADIONUCLIDE STUDY OF A BENIGN
                  MIXED TUMOR

    A.   This is a sonogram of a well-circumscribed mass (black arrow) of the right
parotid gland. The mass was described as a mixed tumor.

    B.   This radionuclide parotid scan shows a photon-deficient area due to a benign
mixed tumor (black arrowhead). (A and B from DelBalso, A., et al: Parotid
masses: Current modes of diagnostic imaging. Oral Surg 54(3):361–363, 1982.)

SONOGRAM OF A MIXED TUMOR; RADIONUCLIDE STUDY OF A BENIGN   **Plate 134**
MIXED TUMOR

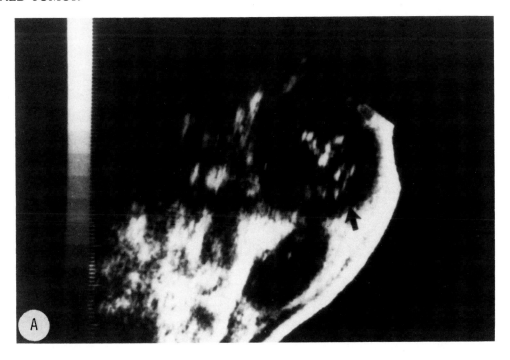

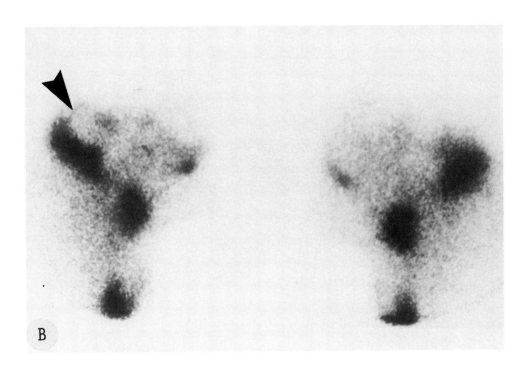

Plate 135   AXIAL CT SCAN OF A SIALOLITH IN THE HILUS; CORONAL CT SCAN OF AN EXPANSILE LESION.

A.   This axial computerized tomogram (CT scan) is a section through the floor of the mouth demonstrating a sialolith (black arrowhead) in the hilus.

B.   Coronal CT scan shows an expansile lesion (black arrowheads) in the right mandible. Note the absence of segments of the medial cortical plate due to previous surgery. (A and B courtesy of Dr. Angelo DelBalso.)

AXIAL CT SCAN OF A SIALOLITH IN THE HILUS; CORONAL CT SCAN OF
AN EXPANSILE LESION.

Plate 135

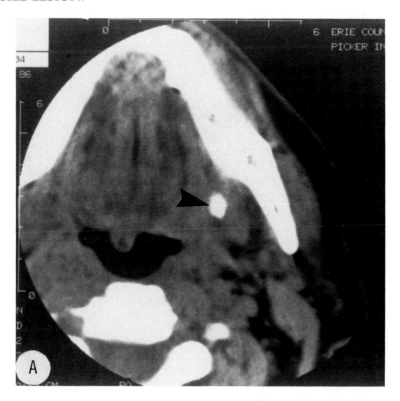

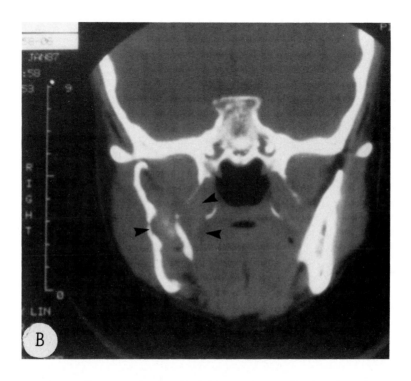

Plate 136 CT SCAN OF A MUCOCELE; AXIAL CT SCAN OF A LE FORT II FRACTURE

A. The area outlined by the white arrowheads is a mucocele arising in the ethmoid sinus. This CT scan shows a marked deformity of the patient's midface.

B. This axial CT scan is taken through the patient's midface. This study demonstrates a Le Fort II fracture. (A and B courtesy of Dr. Angelo DelBalso.)

CT SCAN OF A MUCOCELE; AXIAL CT SCAN OF A LE FORT II FRACTURE   **Plate 136**

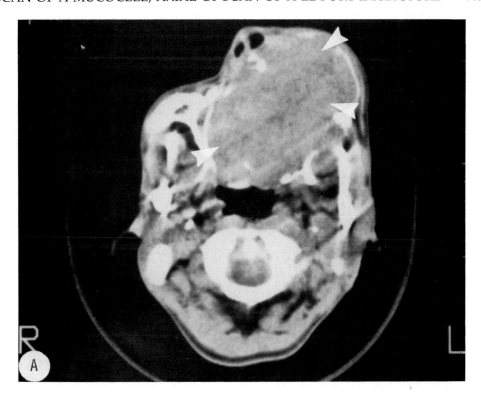

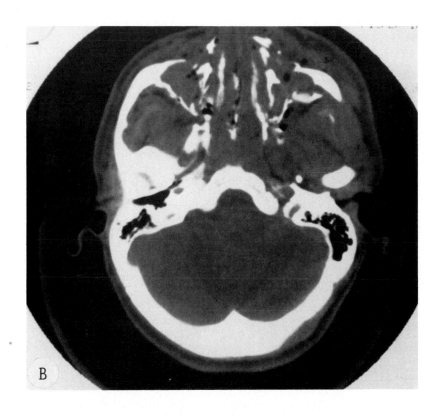

Plate 137   CORONAL CT SCAN OF A VERRUCOUS CARCINOMA; CT SCAN OF A
                     SQUAMOUS CELL CARCINOMA

A.   Direct coronal CT scan through the premaxilla. The study shows a destructive
          lesion destroying the premaxilla and invading the nasal fossa. This lesion was
          described as a verrucous carcinoma of the premaxilla.

B.   CT scan outlining an area of diffuse loss of normal tissue anatomy (black
          arrows). The right half of the tongue was involved, and it should be noted that
          this scan was ordered to rule out a tumor of the submandibular gland. This
          tumor was diagnosed as a squamous cell carcinoma. (A and B courtesy of Dr.
          Angelo DelBalso.)

CORONAL CT SCAN OF A VERRUCOUS CARCINOMA; CT SCAN OF A SQUAMOUS CELL CARCINOMA

Plate 137

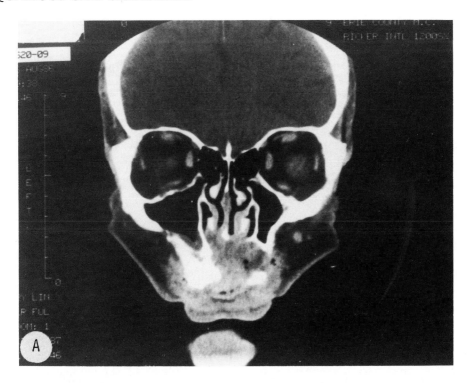

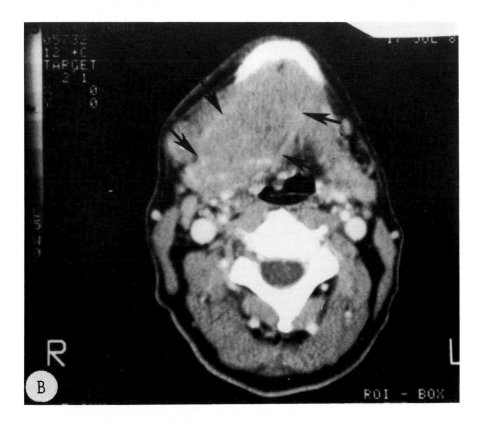

Plate 138   CT SCAN OF A GIANT CELL TUMOR

This CT scan shows a giant cell tumor of the right mandible. The black arrows point to the margin of the tumor. Note the effect of the tumor on the parapharyngeal space (white arrowhead). (Courtesy of Dr. Angelo DelBalso.)

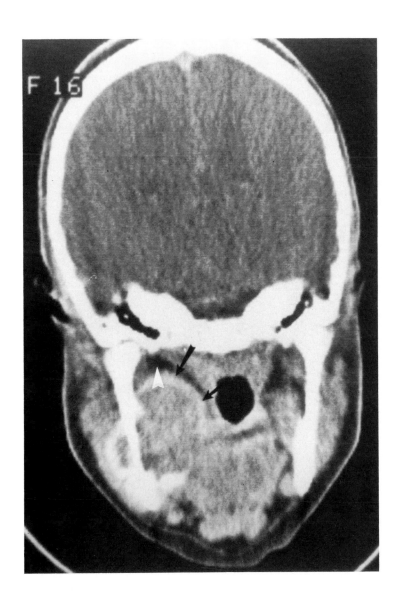

Index